PRAISE FOR TWO MOTHERS, ONE PRAYER

"As the father of two daughters and a son, I can only imagine the heartache of learning that one of my children has cancer. Laura and Laurie have shown incredible fortitude in supporting their daughters. Their story will touch, inspire and provide hope to every parent who loves their children. If you're a parent, be sure you read this book."

Chris Attwood, NY Times Bestselling author of
The Passion Test and Your Hidden Riches

"Beautiful and inspiring! You can feel the love Laura and Laurie have for their daughters. The wonderful relationship they formed to support each other is amazing."

Janet Bray Attwood, New York Times Bestselling Author of
Your Hidden Riches and The Passion Test

"Beautifully written and touching to the core! What these two mothers have endured is both heart-breaking and inspiring. In Two Mothers, One Prayer they show us how they were able to overcome so much with love and grace. They are incredible examples of courage, strength and hope to their daughters and to each of us."

Marci Schimoff, Author of the #1 NY Times Bestsellers
Happy for No Reason, Love For No Reason,
Chicken Soup for the Woman's Soul

"I loved the fact that this book demonstrated that no matter what road the cancer journey may take your family down one must always remain positive and hold on to HOPE with both hands. This book is a must-read for everyone as the lessons and messages conveyed in the book can certainly be applied to any day-to-day life situations."

Coral-Ann Bierer

"Two Mothers One Prayer, is an inspiring story of how people take a tragedy and turn it into an inspiring mission. With Laura's experiences she has created a new outlook on life and parenting. I endorse Laura Lane with this book and any project she pursues in the future in her efforts to helping people and families battle cancer. Any parent needs to read this book, it will inspire to become a better parent."

Dr. Alok Trivedi

"This is not an easy read but it is an inspirational one. I cannot imagine, nor do I want to imagine living through such an ordeal, but if I had to, I would thank God for bringing Celeste and Laura, and Hayley and Laurie into my life. An invaluable resource for parents and their children living with cancer."

Kelly Daniels, Director and Actor

"While reading Two Mothers One Prayer: Facing your child's cancer with Hope, Strength and Courage, I asked myself what did I learn, what message are these two stalwart Mothers are trying so sincerely to convey. The answer I discovered was quite simple, yet profound; the outstretched arms of a Mother in never ending hope for their child is the most perfect example of unconditional love found in this life."

Jeff Roy, PGA Professional and father of 5.

"Heartfelt and moving, this is a book that brings tears, hope, and the presence of beauty and God to the surface of each of us. These two connected families demonstrated the power of community and the inner strength, courage and hope we all can tap into, when and if needed"

Dr. Carrie Rongits, ND Fonthill Naturopathic Clinic

"*Two Mothers, One Prayer*—two moms' moving accounts of their families' childhood cancer journeys told with honesty, love, humour and respect via their shared emails makes for compelling reading."

Susan Kuczynski, OPACC Parent Liaison

"Two Mothers, One Prayer carries the reader on a beautiful journey though the devastating world of childhood cancer. Navigating the day to day struggles with love and courage, inspiring hope on every page."

Christina Rasmussen, Author,
Second Firsts: Live, Laugh and Love Again

"A very moving and powerful book! A must-read for anyone dealing with a life-changing battle with their health."

Dr. Scott Taylor

"Laura, I just finished your book and I have to tell you it is amazing. It is so beautifully written and the actual emails between yourself and Laurie are wonderful. When you spoke about the diagnosis and treatments, I could almost replace Celeste's name with Kelsey; I could relate so well. I really like how you prepared Celeste for the transition and shared that because, really, what do we know about preparing our child for death? I hope that your book can be shared with patients and families in every paediatric oncology ward."

Lana Hill

"I can't put your book down at night. I have been walking around sleep deprived for the past two days. I am halfway through. I feel like I am there with you and Laurie, awaiting test results. The letters that forged your friendship are uplifting and endearing. I will definitely be writing an endorsement for this work and recommending it as a must read . . . Laura, I finished it. I have tears streaming down my face. I already knew the outcome but it did not make it any easier to read. I want you to know, I did not bail on that chapter. I figure if you could go through that and endure it, the least the rest of us can do is travel that journey beside you and not bail. You are the strongest women I know and your heart is one of compassion and purity. Let me think on what way best to express how this book has touched me and why the world needs to hear this story of love and courage and sacrifice."

Sherry Georgeoff, Nurse

"Two courageous women document their heart-wrenching journey through every parent's worst nightmare. If your child is struggling through a serious or terminal illness, please read this book."

Steve Siebold, author, 177 Mental Toughness
Secrets of the World Class

"Any parent whose child has been diagnosed with a life threatening illness will relate to this book!

"As a mother whose 13-year-old daughter was also diagnosed with a brain tumour in February 2011, *Two Mothers, One prayer: Facing Your Child's Cancer with Hope, Strength, and Courage* captivated my heart within seconds of my beginning to read it! The way in which it details the unique loud sounds and magnetic powers of the MRI machine, the deep ache in their hearts when having to say goodbye to their daughters for surgery, the anxiety as they wait for test results, and the overwhelming sense of fear for what lies ahead for their sweet girls brought chills to my soul. It is not by choice that you wish to understand what it truly feels like, but it is because of your own experience that you know exactly what it feels like in those moments. It is that sense of helplessness and fear that connects us so deeply. It was as if they were writing about what I had felt and thought, although they knew nothing about our story.

"When your child is diagnosed with a brain tumour or any life-threatening illness such as cancer, your world as you knew it changes completely, and forever. You would do anything to trade places with your child. It is your worst nightmare and you begin searching and seeking for anyone or anything that will bring you comfort and strength to get you through this life-changing journey. Laura and Laurie certainly found each other in the midst of their search. Living miles apart yet close at heart through sharing the same journey, the women in this book demonstrate one of their many hidden blessings received during this very difficult time.

"For Celeste and Hayley, their courage, bravery, and determination guided them to creating, nurturing, and sharing such a special friendship that only they will fully understand and appreciate.

"It is clear that God knew they needed each other, had special plans for each of them, nurtured their belief of hope through prayer, and created a sisterhood for both girls and their moms that will live on forever.

"We may never understand 'why' this happens to our children. But what this book helps us to understand is that in the midst of the 'why' and the understandable sense of anger, sadness, and despair, there is a greater plan. One too great for us to really understand. However if you can find a way to seek your faith and the willingness to open up your broken heart, there you will find the many hidden blessings offering you comfort, support, hope, and love during your darkest of days."

Rachel, mom to a brave and courageous girl named Janica

Susan ♡ Laura

TWO MOTHERS, ONE PRAYER

Hope Strength
+
Courage

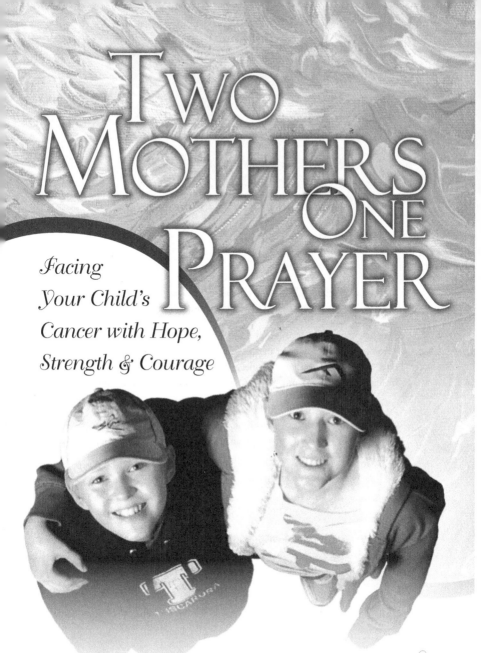

TWO MOTHERS ONE PRAYER

Facing Your Child's Cancer with Hope, Strength & Courage

LAURA LANE &
LAURIE NERSTEN

ULUKAU PUBLISHING
Fonthill, Ontario

Two Mothers One Prayer:
Facing Your Child's Cancer with Hope, Strength & Courage
Copyright © 2015 Ulukau Publishing

Published by Ulukau Publishing
Fonthill, Ontario
Canada

Cover and Interior Design by Imagine! Studios, LLC
www.ArtsImagine.com

ISBN: 978-0-9876967-2-4

First Ulukau Publishing printing: February 2015

Dedicated to our two beautiful girls,

Celeste and Hayley,

and our wonderful husbands,

Matthew and Anthony,

who supported us through everything, as well as to our
other most awesome children:

Desiree, Connlan, and Grayson
Taylor and Matthew

CONTENTS

Foreword . . . . *xv*

PART ONE

Chapter 1 Introduction 3

Chapter 2 Celeste's Story 11

Chapter 3 Hayley's Story 23

PART TWO

Chapter 4 Getting to Know One Another 37

Chapter 5 A Friendship Blossoms 51

Chapter 6 Supporting Each Other 71

Chapter 7 The Road to Recovery 111

PART THREE

Chapter 8   Reach Out and Connect 151

Chapter 9   Reflect 159

Chapter 10   Express 167

Chapter 11   Love 175

PART FOUR

Chapter 12   How Do You Cope When the Worst
             Happens? 185

Chapter 13   Hope, Strength, and Courage 213

Recommended Resources 219

Our Gratitude List! 221

About the Authors 225

FOREWORD

Bad things happen to all of us at one time or another. Anyone who has senses—who sees, hears, feels, smells, tastes—has had to endure something difficult, something trying, something so painful that it seems as if the world has ended. On Monday September 12th 2011 our son in law called to tell us that our beautiful daughter Summer had been whisked to hospital. Our whole family and numerous friends came together to help us and care for three of our grandchildren, while we gathered in the emergency waiting room, awaiting the results of the scans. As the doctor approached, she shared with us that Summer had two brain tumours and she would be required to undergo surgery.

Over the next few days and weeks we were in awe of her resilient spirit as she harnessed this adversity and turned it into a launching pad for doing good. She inspired my wife Sherry and I and we in turn put all of our focus on remaining positive and surrounding her with positive people and positive thoughts. Gratitude comes from grace and grace means "Divine gift." We were so grateful for the faithful people from all over the world who prayed for our cherished daughter Summer. It meant more than words can describe, all except one word of course—Gratitude. Our family received such a huge outpouring of love and we were blessed to be reminded of all the good in the world and what was most important—family and love and the importance of keeping a divine perspective.

At that time a friend pointed out to me that a mothers prayers are heard before all others because the strength and velocity in which they are sent is second only to God's love for us. I watched as my wife knelt in prayer for her daughter and how my daughter knelt in prayer to be able to stay a little long on this earth to continue to raise her beautiful children. Theirs was the same prayer as Laura Lane and Laurie Nersten had for their respective daughters, Celeste and Hayley.

When I met Laura Lane in 2010 through my friend Bob Proctor and again this year as we spent time together at my Genshai Life Mastery retreat, I was struck by her beautiful capacity to love and trust in God and her passion for her daughter Celeste. Passion means sacred suffering and a willingness to suffer for who and what you love. Here is a valiant mother, an inspired, sweet soul, full of incredible wisdom and insights, who was willing to dedicated all of herself to her child and also have empathy and compassion, to share in the suffering of another family and walk the path with Laurie and her daughter Hayley in the midst of her own difficult struggles.

Theirs is such a beautiful story. You will find as you read their story of love and hope and passion for their daughters, it will inspire you—breathe new life into you. They have truly become pathfinders, paving the way for you and your family, mapping out a route for you to follow on your journey of childhood cancer. As you follow them on their journey you will feel their love and empathy; their willingness to walk the path with you.

We all have a story—and Laura's journey and story of spiritual strength will touch, open and heal your heart.

Kevin Hall, Author,
Aspire: Discovering Your Purpose Through the Power of Words

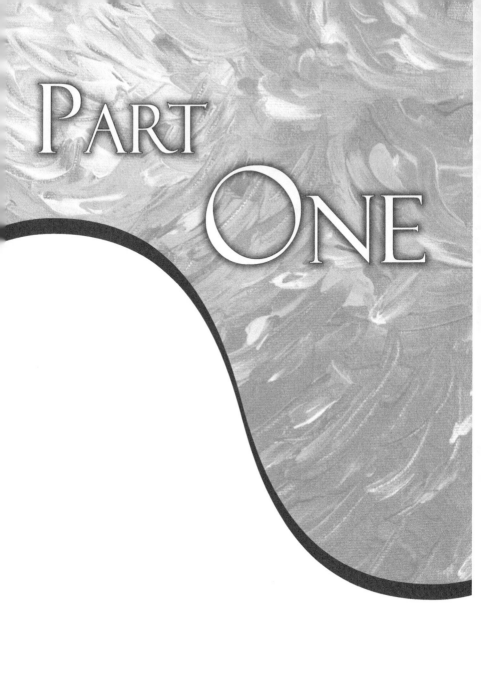

PART ONE

"There is no medicine like hope, no tonic more powerful than belief that every trauma has a solution. The ability to hope allows us to face the trials of daily life."

LEO BUSCAGLIA

Chapter 1

INTRODUCTION

"I am so happy and grateful that my daughter Celeste has had a miraculous recovery and her brain tumour has shrunk completely and has disappeared. I am so happy and grateful for family and friends all over the world who have prayed and fasted and visualized a full, complete, and speedy recovery for Celeste. I am so happy and grateful now that all the prayers and visualizations for Celeste have effectively restored her to complete health."

Written on a small notepad at midnight
Thursday, February 24, 2011

L ittle did I know that night of the incredible journey our family was about to embark on and the impact it would have on thousands of lives. I will forever remember writing that note. I will forever remember that day. I will forever remember all the details of the events that occurred over the next two years.

At 4 o'clock in the afternoon on Thursday, February 24, 2011, my husband, Matt, and I had just picked up my 6-year-old son, Grayson, from school. Climbing back into our car, I scrambled to grab my ringing cell phone. It was Michelle, my children's stepmother. She hurriedly informed me that Celeste, my 12-year-old daughter, was in the emergency department of the Children's Hospital in London, Ontario.

Celeste had been having bad headaches, and we had a doctor's appointment coming, but when she started developing double vision that morning, Michelle, a neurology resident, took Celeste to see her doctor that day. He immediately sent Celeste over to the emergency department. They did a CAT scan and an MRI was scheduled.

Michelle announced, "Celeste has to have emergency neuro [brain] surgery tonight."

"We're on our way!" I said. I was in shock.

London is a two-hour drive from my home in Niagara. I began making calls to family and friends to let them know what was happening and to request their help arranging a priesthood blessing for Celeste before her surgery, a place to stay for Matt and Grayson while I stayed at the hospital with Celeste, and any other help we might need while staying in London.

Matt and I had been in the midst of a celebration getaway at a hotel in Niagara Falls, a gift from my parents to celebrate my fortieth birthday and our seventh wedding anniversary coming up that weekend. We raced back to the hotel, packed our bags, cancelled our dinner reservation, and informed the hotel we would have to check out a day early.

It was all so surreal.

When we arrived at the hospital, Celeste's father, David, himself a doctor of child psychiatry, met us and quickly explained that the CAT scan and MRI had found a large mass (3 centimetres x 3 centimetres x 3 centimetres) near her pineal gland, close to the brain stem. It was blocking the flow of her brain fluid, which was building up, and that pressure was causing the headaches and double vision.

The surgery would relieve the pressure and the doctors hoped to get a biopsy of the tumour to assess if it was benign or cancerous. They had no way of knowing how long it had been growing. David then informed me that Celeste didn't know and that he didn't want to tell her until after we knew something concrete, until we had a firm diagnosis and treatment plan.

Armed with all this new information, I was taken to Celeste in her little children's room in the ER. How do you cope when you have just been told your daughter has a tumour and she doesn't know about it? How do you put on a calm face for your precious daughter?

You just do.

I was emotionally exhausted before I even stepped into her room, yet adrenaline and focusing on what needed to be done kept me marching on. We arranged for the bishop to give her a blessing before her scheduled surgery at 9:30 p.m. Celeste was tired, medicated to deal with the pain in her head, and she had a patch on her eye to help with the double vision.

Armed with her Pooh Bear, blanket, and Winnie the Pooh movie, Celeste waited for her surgery. Grayson climbed into bed with her and cuddled. When it was time to head to surgery, I went with Celeste to pre-op.

Celeste did so well, taking everything in stride. We joked with the nurses as they gave her meds to make her sleepy and off they wheeled her down the hallway. Now, looking back, I don't know how I was so strong to watch them take her away, my baby girl.

If I could have, I would have stayed holding her hand during the whole surgery.

It was a long, tiring wait in a cold, empty waiting room. Both Michelle and I tried to sleep on the tiny bench seating, to no avail. The surgery went well and, around midnight, we were ushered into post-op to wait for Celeste to wake and then finally have something to eat and drink. She hadn't eaten all day, poor thing.

The incision was about three inches long and she had a dozen stitches. They had very carefully shaved just that area of her head but it was all bandaged up now with a tube protruding from the incision to help drain the fluid. The tube was connected to a bag to monitor, measure, and collect the fluid. Every time she lay down or sat up, they had to adjust the bag to keep it level with her head.

When Celeste was finally in her own room in the children's ward, my adrenaline was gone. The pullout chair turned into a tiny single bed. As I settled down to sleep, I focused all my thoughts on visualizing Celeste well again. I started planning in my mind how to recruit all our family and friends all over the world to pray for her complete recovery.

My fervent prayer was for a miracle. I had just spent the previous year learning from Bob Proctor, personal growth and development expert, about how the mind works and how fear is generated by ignorance. I was determined to stay focused on the positive, arm myself with knowledge, and ground myself with faith and gratitude.

I felt calm. I fell asleep.

———

Five hundred miles away in the United States, in New Jersey, there was another 12-year-old girl and her family dealing with the exact same situation. Hayley had been on a much longer journey to discovering the source of her symptoms. Over a period of six months, doctors told Hayley's mom, Laurie, that it was possibly everything from kidney issues or tumours on her adrenal to a thyroid problem or anxiety.

They had performed every blood and urine test imaginable, CT scans, MRI scans, MIBG scans, and ultrasounds, but it wasn't until Laurie finally took Hayley to another paediatrician that he recognized the double vision and her eye beginning to turn inward that he sent them directly to the emergency room. Within an hour, Hayley had been diagnosed with a tumour on her pineal gland, just at the top of the brain stem. She was then admitted to the ICU and scheduled the next day for neurosurgery to relieve the pressure of the hydrocephalus (fluid build-up in the brain).

Laurie and I, hundreds of miles of apart, shared a journey that no mother ever dreams of, and we had no idea then that we would share each other's journeys. We didn't learn of each other until three months later. This book chronicles our stories and how it is our wish that our story will help another mother when she gets the devastating news that her child has cancer.

One of our daughters survived. One did not.

During the days, weeks, and months following surgery, the learning curve, for both Laurie and me, was extremely steep. We stepped into a new world of hospitals, doctors, nurses, support staff, new terminology, new procedures and tests, and information and emotional overload as we tried to prepare ourselves for everything we needed to know and do to best help our little girls. There isn't a manual for being a parent when your bundle of joy is first placed in your arms, and there certainly isn't a manual on how to cope when you receive the heart-wrenching news that your beautiful child has cancerous cells growing in her body. You only hope that all your life experiences thus far can help you deal with the difficulties that lie ahead.

As two mothers who have used every ounce of hope, strength, and courage necessary to help our daughters bravely face their treatments and adjust to life as cancer survivors, we wrote this book for you to share how we supported each other as one daughter learned her cancer had become terminal. We would like to share with you some of the things we did to cope during the long days and nights—through surgeries, diagnosis, treatments, and the aftermath.

We share the gift of the friendship that developed between me, Laura, the mother of Celeste, and my friend Laurie, the mother of Hayley. As the girls started their chemotherapy treatments, a rare and special friendship blossomed between us as we shared with each other the same journey of faith, hope, prayer, and desire to witness a miracle of healing for both girls. We strengthened and supported each other on low days and praised the miracles on good days.

We communicated by email nearly every day and when time allowed via Skype and phone. Our personal story is shared here through some of our email exchanges. You will bear witness to a friendship and love that blossomed during the long summer of 2011.

The following chapters include an introduction to Celeste, an introduction to Hayley, some of our emails, and what we have learned through it all.

Our main objective is to share how to find hope, strength, and courage. As we reflect on what it took to get through those long difficult months, we share tools, resources, and lessons we learned in order to help other parents and loved ones face the reality of caring for a child with cancer with hope, strength, and courage.

In sharing the personal details of our stories, we wish to help you on your journey. Our experiences taught us what we convey to you: the importance of:

- Reaching out to the resources and family and friends around you for support

- Connecting with God/spirit, friends, and other parents going through the same thing

- Reflecting on the present situation through reading, prayer, meditation—arming yourself with knowledge to better learn how to help your child

- Expressing the torrent of emotions that will come up by journaling, talking it out, crying, and being creative

- Loving yourself, your family, God/spirit, and, most importantly, your child.

For you to get through your journey with hope, strength, and courage, it will be crucial for you reach out, connect, reflect, express, and love. That is what drove us to write this book.

It has not been easy to write this book and yet it has been healing.

All we can do is share what we have done and hope that it helps you.

Chapter 2

CELESTE'S STORY

Celeste is my second child. Her older sister is Desiree, and she has two younger brothers, Connlan and Grayson. Celeste was 12 at the time of her diagnosis and had been living with her dad and stepmother for the previous six months. She had been adjusting to her new home and school when she started having headaches, really bad headaches, that woke her up in the middle of the night.

I had been worried that she was being plagued with migraines and wondered how she would cope with that through her teenage years. There was no way I could be prepared for the news that it was cancer.

Celeste was born June 8, 1998, two weeks early after I had spent a month in the hospital on bed rest because of pre-term labor. Six weeks later we were back in hospital. My tiny little baby had developed pertussis syndrome, coughing until she threw up. I slept on a cot next to her crib in her hospital room, still nursing her every two to three hours. Poor little thing, at night I would have her sleep on my chest so I would know immediately when she started coughing and threw up. That way I could keep her from choking on it and could clean her up right away. That meant she was throwing up on me, repeatedly, but I didn't care. I had already decided that, as her Mummy, I would do anything for her. Back at home, I quickly learned that she had a need to be held. It was as if Celeste had a quota she needed filled every day. If I didn't hold her enough during the day because she was in her swing or car seat then she would cry at night until she had been held enough.

After I finally clued in to her needs, she became a permanent attachment, being carried around in the sling all day so I could get some sleep at night. But it wasn't a hardship. I loved carrying her. I'm glad she insisted in her own little way.

Twelve years later I became a permanent fixture in her hospital room through all the chemotherapy and procedures. I was always climbing into her bed and holding her, cuddling during the day while we watched the television show *iCarly* and holding her until she fell asleep at night.

Celeste was always a very strong-willed child, making her wishes known. She could give her Mummy a run for her money! I told her now that her strong will would help get her through all her treatments.

I remember that first night in the hospital after Celeste came out of surgery. I helped her have a drink and a Popsicle before she could be taken up to a room. I was so proud of my strong daughter. As we transferred her to the children's ward and put her to bed, I knew we needed more than strong will to help her get through this. We needed people's prayers, all the positive energy we could get.

I wrote out a special note on my Facebook page:

Dear family and friends,

I am writing this today Feb 25th 2011 from the children's hospital in London, Ontario. I ask for your prayers for Celeste. I am posting this as a note because Desiree and Connlan, as of today, do not know the full extent of Celeste's condition, nor does she. I don't want to scare them until we know exactly what sort of treatments Celeste will require.

Last night Celeste had an emergency operation to relieve the fluid that has built up in her brain. (She knows this much.) But the reason she has fluid build-up is because a tumour has developed. We do not have results back on the status of her tumour. She will require another operation at Sick Kids in Toronto to do a biopsy. After that it may require radiation therapy or an operation to shrink or remove the tumour.

The key thing is we want the tumour gone. I am asking for your prayers, fasting and visualizing the tumour shrinking and disappearing completely. I know that prayers work, that the collective efforts of many to visualize and pray for an outcome have miraculous effects.

If you can please add her name (Celeste Ebony Claire Templeman) to prayer lists and prayer circles, I would greatly appreciate it. Please feel free to post messages for Celeste on this note and I will share your messages with her. Thanks you for all your love, support and encouragement.

With gratitude and faith, Laura Lane

That was the first of countless posts I made to Facebook over the next two years. The support we received was overwhelming. I would keep people up to date and it helped me feel connected.

> Thank you, everyone. Celeste had a good day today. She had a long-needed nap. The fluids continue to drain, which has alleviated the headaches and back pain. Her appetite is returning to normal and she has just spent all evening watching *iCarly*! She finds it easier to watch with an eye patch on until the double vision goes away. We're hoping her eyesight should be back to normal in a day or two. She spent the morning with Grayson cuddled up with her and the evening with Desiree and Connlan. I will be spending the night here with her again tonight.

> *26 February 2011*

Those first few days in London were the hardest, scrambling to find people to help, trying to figure out our needs, learning new medical lingo and procedures, not knowing what to tell Celeste and her siblings, sleeping—barely—on a cot at the end of her bed, waiting to hear when they would have a bed for her in Toronto.

> Celeste had a good night. She's watching Saturday morning cartoons right now and, great news, we're going to Sick Kids in TO this morning. A bed opened up last night. Thank you for your prayers everyone!

> *26 February 2011*

Before we left her room in London, Celeste was in good spirits, making jokes about her dad. Then we had to move her onto another gurney to travel by ambulance to Toronto. I held her hand,

14

and tried to make her feel as comfortable as possible. It was all so surreal. The paramedics had never been to Sick Kids in Toronto and were driving around trying to figure out what entrance to go to. The building takes up a whole city block in downtown Toronto and we eventually found our way. Celeste was patient through it all.

> Thanks everyone! We made it to Toronto Sick Kids Hospital safely. Celeste is resting and watching a movie. I will be giving her all the messages written out on sticky notes to decorate her room—surrounding her in LOVE!

26 February 2011

Celeste had to be watched for twenty-four hours in a four-bed ward monitored constantly by nursing staff before she was finally assigned to her own private room. In the ward there was only room for a reclining chair and only one parent could be with Celeste at a time. Once she was in her own room, we could have two visitors at a time and the couch seating turned into a bed for whichever parent was staying over that night.

She had visits from aunts and uncles, grandmas and grandpas, and calls from family in Utah as we learned we would have to wait a couple of more days until her test results came back.

Celeste filled her days and late nights with hours upon hours of *iCarly*. I would climb into bed with her and watch the episodes on her laptop. She wanted me to watch the whole season with her. It was such precious time together. She would fall asleep in my arms, and then I would crawl off into the little daybed on the other side of the tiny room.

There was a small closet in the room, as well as three drawers under the daybed. A long shelf provided room for books and displaying get-well cards above the daybed. The room was a weird pink-peach color that we only sort of got used to. Across from her bed was a white board used for leaving messages. The nurses would write their name at the change of every shift, so we would know whom to ask for if we had to buzz the nurse's station for help. Every day Celeste would wake up to the new row of sticky notes on her walls, announcing who else was praying for her and sending well wishes. Our wall of love was starting to get noticed by the nurses and other staff.

Celeste's eyesight was getting better, but until the double vision cleared up completely she would need to keep wearing her eye patch. Her MRIs were often scheduled late at night and we would get back to her room sometimes at two o'clock in the morning or later.

She was such a trooper. We would just stay up watching *iCarly* until it was time to be taken through all the confusing back hallways down to the basement radiology department. They would give me a little locker to put my valuables in: cell phone, rings, and pens, anything that might have metal on it. They let me keep my glasses on if they fit snugly and when the MRI would start with its loud pulsing vibration I would feel the snap of my bra pulling away from me for the duration of the procedure. It would snap back onto my shoulder as soon as the machine turned off. Such a powerful machine. I'm glad the wires on my teeth were securely cemented in place so they wouldn't pop out of my mouth and zing across the room.

With all the MRIs and tests, we were getting to know the hospital quite well, being wheeled around the back hallways at all times of the day and night. Celeste was patient through it all. She began putting together her bravery bead necklace. She would add beads for every poke and procedure and surgery she was enduring. Her biggest excitement was phone calls from her friends back home.

We finally had a date scheduled for the next surgery. The biopsy would be Thursday, March 3, and we would have to wait a week for the results.

On the day of her surgery, we had a long wait in a huge waiting room filled with parents. It was a complicated system to keep track of where our child was at each stage and when we could finally be with her in recovery. I had to do it again—watch her being wheeled away for her second surgery in a week, kissing her again, making sure she had her Pooh Bear and blanket, everything labelled so as not to be lost.

Then finally being allowed back in recovery, holding her hand, helping her to come back to consciousness, more juice and Popsicles, and back to her room again. It was the hardest thing in the world.

Fortunately the surgery went well. Life went back to our new normal. Friends and family coming to visit. Grayson would climb up into bed with Celeste and they would watch TV together all day. When Desy and Connlan came by, they played hours of video games together. A wonderful friend from Toronto came by with homemade chocolate cupcakes that disappeared oh-so-quickly. Dan will forever be known now as Cupcake Dan to our family!

Plans were made for the drain tube to come out after another CAT scan. The results were good, all her "brain juice" as we called it was draining well, but they wanted to keep the tube in a little longer until she wasn't seeping through her incision any longer. This became more of our new normal: medical terms, procedures, tests, and leaky brain juice.

Then came the results of the biopsy and her diagnosis.

The doctors squeezed us into a little room with the social worker and head nurse—myself; my husband, Matt; stepmom, Michelle; and her dad, David, listening via conference call from his office in London. The doctor told us the diagnosis and treatment plan. As silent tears rolled down my face, my heart broke for my little girl and all she was going to have to go through. Now we had to bravely go back to her room to inform her, help her understand her diagnosis and all the treatments she would be required to undergo over the next six to eight months.

Telling my daughter that she had cancer was the hardest thing I have ever had to do.

Celeste would be participating in the St. Jude's protocol. It was the best option they could offer her. She had the best neurosurgeon in Canada performing her surgery. Her tumour was in such a tricky spot to gain access to that he later asked permission to create a model of her brain based on her MRIs to be used by medical students so they could practice and gain more experience dealing with these types of tumours. It was reassuring to us that right across the street was the Brain Tumour Research Centre building. Now her team of physicians would consist of the best doctors in London and Toronto. She would be treated in London for her radiation and Toronto for her high-dose chemotherapy and stem cell rescue.

Later that day we posted to friends and family:

> We now have a diagnosis for Celeste. She has pineoblastoma, a malignant cancer located near the pineal gland and also in her spinal cord. Doctors wish to treat her with six weeks of radiation and four to six months of chemotherapy. Please continue to pray for her and visualize these tumours being surrounded in white light and melting the tumours just like the sun melts an ice cube.

Starting tomorrow, Celeste will have some smaller procedures to go through before the radiation starts in three weeks. We are hoping that she gets to go home tomorrow afternoon and just come back as an outpatient for the other procedures next week and the following week. Thank you so much for your prayers and support.

Celeste was so anxious to go home, to go back to school and get back to work. She was so disappointed that her teacher wouldn't send any homework for her to do while she was in the hospital. She would be heading home just as everyone was getting out to enjoy March break. We could have a few days together at home before it was back to appointments in London and Toronto.

The day she was released was a busy day with three different tests. Her stitches and incisions were healing well. We had the weekend to spend time together as a family, including pancakes, bowling, a new haircut, time with Grandad, then church and family movies, and then it was time go back to her dad's house in London. That was another very difficult day for me, sending her back to her dad's, not being able to spend every moment looking after her as I had in the hospital. It became a recurring heartache.

Watching her go, I refocused myself, redoubling my efforts to enlist the help of as many people as possible to visualize and pray for a miracle. We wanted people to visualize the tumour shrinking and the doctors seeing the tumour disappear on the MRI. We organized a special prayer, asking everyone—thousands of people—to all pray for Celeste at a pre-arranged time: Sunday March 20, at nine o'clock in the evening, Eastern time, or whatever time that was in their part of the world.

We drove to London to meet her new doctor there and do more blood tests. Her double vision had improved so much so that she didn't need to wear the eye patch anymore. A week later we went back to Sick Kids in Toronto. She had a femoral line put in so that they could perform a stem cell harvest. The procedure was supposed to take seven hours a day for two, three, or four days, however long it took to get the needed number of cells to harvest and freeze to use later. She was such a trooper. She played Nancy Drew games on the computer and ate spring rolls and French fries. At the end of that first day, they gave us the good news: They were able to successfully harvest all the cells they needed in one shot! Not only did we know that she's one awesome little girl, but we knew that the group prayer had brought us another beautiful miracle.

Celeste finally went back to school after that procedure. She was so excited to see her friends again and the whole school was thrilled to have her back. She came home reporting how she was practically mobbed by everyone. They all wanted to tell her how happy they were to see her.

Things returned to a semblance of normalcy in the intervening weeks before she started radiation in London. Celeste had another CAT scan and they fit her for her mask and tattooed dots on her face and body to mark where they would line everything up to keep her perfectly straight while radiating her brain and spine.

Four days before starting her first radiation treatment, Celeste and I attended a large church youth activity for all the 12- to 18-year-old young women in greater Toronto area. She received a very special priesthood blessing that night, praying that her tumours would shrink and she would have the strength to endure the treatments she was about to go through.

I let Celeste know that as soon as she had that first treatment, she would now officially qualify to have a special wish granted by the Make-A-Wish Foundation. I asked her what her wish would be.

She wanted to meet Celine Dion or be in an episode of *Doctor Who* and meet the whole cast.

Celeste had a rough go of it the first week, throwing up quite a bit, not eating much, and needing an IV for fluids by the end of the week. She felt much better on Saturday and was able to participate in the Brain Tumour Foundation of Canada's 2.5-kilometer Spring Sprint. She raised $1,250 out of the total $2,000 that her class team raised. The principal and a huge group of kids from school came out to cheer her on! It tired her out, but it didn't slow her down.

For the next four weeks she seemed to sail right through her treatments. It wasn't until the last week that she seemed to be waning a bit, but then treatments were finally over and she would have a month break before she had to start chemotherapy in July.

Celeste did lose her hair but had fun alternating between being a blond and a brunette until the wigs just became too itchy and she stopped wearing them altogether. She donned her baseball cap and just didn't care! She was my awesome little trooper. We were sure she could do anything and knew we were going to see miracles.

That first miracle came July 6, 2011. We had the results of the MRI: Her tumor had shrunk 84 percent and the smaller cyst had shrunk 70 percent. Her lumbar puncture had come back with no trace of cancer cells in her spine. We were ecstatic!

And by now we were sharing our news, the good and not so good, with our new friends, Hayley and her mom, Laurie.

"I learned that courage was not the absence of fear, but the triumph over it. The brave man is not he who does not feel afraid, but he who conquers that fear."

NELSON MANDELA

Chapter 3

HAYLEY'S STORY
(From her mom, Laurie's, perspective)

Hayley was always a thin little girl, but at age 12, she started looking particularly skinny. When she would get dressed, I noticed that I could actually see her ribs. During her scheduled physical, I mentioned it to her paediatrician. He said that Hayley had grown a couple of inches, so it was probably just a growth spurt and her weight would catch up.

I accepted his answer, to some extent, because she was very active with soccer and other activities and I wanted to quell my maternal sensor that was entering worry mode.

Hayley had never really had a huge appetite, but I began to notice that she was eating less and less. It was a battle to get her to eat during meals, but she seemed to have an appetite for junk food.

My mommy heart was unsettled, but I wanted to believe it was just normal pre-teen changes.

Hayley began to have what I called "episodes," that included a racing heart, skin pallor, and weakness. Her older sister, Taylor, was lying on the couch with her one evening and mentioned that she could feel Hayley's heart beating out of her chest. I called the paediatrician the next morning. This began the long process of trying to determine what was wrong with my baby.

Test after test proved normal. Nothing could be found through blood tests or examinations, yet we knew what was going on was not normal.

After additional blood tests, it was determined that Hayley's potassium level was low, her calcium was high, and her parathyroid hormone level was high.

I contacted the Children's Hospital of Philadelphia (CHOP) and spoke with the endocrinology department. Hayley was found to have a very high heart rate—twice the normal range for a 12-year-old girl. She was also found to have dangerously high blood pressure.

She began taking atenolol and amlodipine to get these levels under control. We had no idea then that tests and doctors and rattling off the names of meds would become our new normal.

Hayley was given several more tests, including an ultrasound of her thyroid, CT scans from her neck down, twenty-four-hour urine tests, and an MIBG test. The MIBG is an imaging test that uses a scanner and radioactive substance called a tracer. This test is used to find or confirm the existence of tumours.

All the tests came back normal, except for the MIBG test.

This test showed an increased uptake on both of her adrenal glands. I contacted the endocrinology department again and asked for an appointment. I was thankful, yet horrified, when the division chief of the department was the person who called me back for an appointment. He said he had reviewed Hayley's online CHOP records and wanted to see her. Of course, panic set in.

My husband, Anthony, is a much calmer person than I am. We have completely different philosophies. He feels that we shouldn't worry until we have confirmation to panic. I, on the other hand, have always gone into panic mode at the hint of something wrong.

I knew that Anthony was a little worried because he took the day off and came to the appointment with me. We were greeted by the division chief as well as an attending and a fellow physician. We were told that from Hayley's tests, they believed that she had a syndrome called MEN2A (multiple endocrine neoplasia type 2), which is a group of disorders associated with tumours of the endocrine system. The doctors would need to confirm this through genetic testing, but they were 90 percent to 95 percent positive that she had this rare condition.

The doctors told us that if she did indeed have this condition, the treatment would involve removing both of her adrenal glands as well as her thyroid gland.

I felt entitled to panic now. *What?! What do you mean? This is crazy!* We were told that her adrenals were probably cancerous or pre-cancerous and that Hayley's thyroid would more than likely turn cancerous at some point.

Fear and disbelief set in.

The doctors wanted to admit her to the hospital on Christmas Eve to prepare for surgery. We were told that because of her low weight (she now weighed just 64 pounds—even at only 5 feet tall, that was much too thin), her high heart rate, and her high blood pressure, no surgeon would perform this surgery until everything was under control.

We convinced the doctors to allow her to go into the hospital the day after Christmas so we could at least enjoy our holiday with our baby and the rest of our family before our hospital stay of at least one month.

Yes, we were entering a new world. Everything as we knew it would never be the same.

After genetic testing, her doctors were surprised that she did not have MEN2A. They were completely baffled. We didn't know what to feel. It was a relief, I suppose, but my daughter was sick and no one could find out what was going on with her. So many tests and no real conclusions. Not knowing does not ease the worry. In many ways, not knowing what is wrong is harder to handle than knowing what you are up against.

Hayley continued to have strange episodes, which included insomnia and hallucinations. She would start telling stories that were completely crazy as well as repeating commercials from television. She was not eating, she was not sleeping, and she was not herself. We did not know what to do, so we brought her to the hospital and insisted on being admitted.

After a weeklong stay at CHOP, we were basically told that nothing was wrong with Hayley except severe anxiety and that I was treating her like a baby. After everything we had gone through, the entire battery of tests Hayley had endured, the near-surgery at Christmas, and now to be told to go home and toughen up, that she was "fine;" it was unreal.

I felt maybe I, too, was now having hallucinations.

We were told by numerous psychologists and psychiatrists that we should send her to school and that she needed to start eating. They placed an NG feeding tube down her nose and told her that she needed to behave like a 12-year-old.

I was irate and told them that I didn't care what they thought of us, but that no 12-year-old girl has high blood pressure, a high heart rate, and hallucinates. They did not know what to say to us. They refused to write a note for her to take some time off from school. I was at my wit's end. Frustration, anger, despair, confusion made up the cocktail swirling in my gut. I knew that something was wrong. I knew my baby was not just acting like a baby. I knew that telling her to "grow up and act her age" was not the cure. I knew there was something and they wouldn't listen to me. It was maddening.

As we were leaving the hospital, Hayley's eyes started to cross. We were told this was just anxiety. We were up against the proverbial brick wall. They offered no solution, and even more painful, no compassion.

Against our better judgment, we allowed Hayley to go to school the next day, but after two classes, I drove to the school and removed her from class. My heart knew we had to get to the bottom of what was wrong with her.

I drove straight to her paediatrician's office and demanded to see a different paediatrician. God definitely guided us, and we were blessed to see one of the only paediatricians in the office that we had never met before. He took one look at Hayley and told me to never let anyone tell me that this was normal for someone with anxiety. He said she was not suffering from anxiety, that she was very sick and I was to drive her immediately to the emergency room.

Within a half hour of arriving at the hospital that day, February 9, 2011, a CT scan revealed our worst fears.

Hayley had a brain tumour and was admitted to the paediatric intensive care unit (PICU).

Two days later, she had ETV surgery to relieve the pressure from the fluid in her brain, which was causing her sleep issues and her crossed eyes. Her full craniotomy and partial resection was performed on February 14. After the surgery, her blood pressure and heart rate went immediately to normal. On February 17, we were given the devastating news that her tumour was cancerous and had spread to her spine. She would require radiation and chemotherapy for her pineoblastoma—her brain tumour.

The panic subsided into a low-grade fear and dread, but for the most part we were too busy to focus on the fear. We now had a diagnosis, and, although it was dreadful and devastating to learn my baby had a brain tumour, I had hope that, now that we knew what was wrong, the doctors could provide the right treatment to bring my daughter out of this nightmare.

The initial days were trying in new ways. It's hard enough to absorb the news mentally and emotionally, but the body is fighting and it is so tiring, on every level.

After the first surgery in February, Hayley had to undergo a three-hour MRI on her spine the next day. We tried to focus on the immediate needs of the day, like loading Hayley up with calories. Facing another five-hour surgery meant she needed to "prepare" and I had to prepare myself for the range (and sometimes rage) of emotions.

There was so much waiting. So much wondering. So many "what ifs."

I kept busy taking care of Hayley and using prayer to keep my mind from careening down the path of negativity.

Small blessings became the stronghold for our family. The morning after the surgery, Anthony sat at her bedside watching her sleep. He was reassured to see her so peaceful, that was so different from the tornado sleep pattern that we had become used to.

As he prayed asking God to watch over her and comfort her, Hayley began to moan in her sleep. She normally would not be calmed no matter what anyone else would say or do until I sat with her and held her hand.

This morning, Anthony took her hand and, for the first time, she stopped moaning for Mom and went back to sleep. He accepted that answer to prayer and was thankful for another small blessing.

Hayley's first days in the hospital set PICU visitor attendance records. Friends, cousins, a steady stream of aunts and uncles—everyone popped in to wish Hayley well.

Anthony was called down to the security office. Not sure what it was about, he expected to be reprimanded for the crowds in the room, but instead was surprised to see a supervisor on walkie-talkie with a gorilla at her side. Someone had sent Hayley a gorilla-gram!

Apparently no one in Philadelphia knew what to do with a singing gorilla, and there was some concern a gorilla with a big red heart walking through the halls of a children's hospital would strike fear into the hearts of sick children. Anthony spent a bit of time in a discussion at the security office devising a plan of how to get a gorilla up to the seventh floor without arousing suspicion. He accompanied the gorilla, a security guard, and a child life representative through the back way and up the service elevator to Hayley's room. It was quite a sight and Hayley was quite surprised.

We focused on our blessings. We covered her room in red hearts. We prayed and read scripture. Even the chaplain at the hospital said he had never seen a little girl so happy before surgery. Hayley had put her trust in the Lord.

As I write this, I recall the pendulum swing of emotions. Knowing we were in God's hands kept us going. I also remember the long nights of Hayley crying in pain. The itching. The facial swelling. The throwing up. The incredible and seemingly incessant discomforts. Most people know cancer leads to hair loss and they think that is hard. Those who are in it, those of you reading this, know that is the least of it.

That said, we are forever grateful to Hayley's friends who had their ponytails cut off for Hayley in the Locks of Love program. Everyone looks beautiful with short hair! And Hayley was deeply touched when her Uncle Keith shaved his head to show his solidarity with her.

I continued to keep my trust in the Lord. We also had faith in our medical team—the oncology department, the endocrinology doctors, the nurses—and our amazing friends and family. We had, and have, a wonderful network of support.

We knew that we were not in control. We knew that truly the doctors were not in control. Only our Lord is in control.

My prayers would change. Most days I would ask for just a bit of good news. A tiny ray of hope to keep my positivity afloat. Hayley was so delicate—my baby, my little angel. No mother ever imagines she will have to watch her child endure so much. There were many tough days and many grueling nights. I was at her side constantly. She barely let me get away to go to the bathroom or get a drink. I knew I needed to be her rock.

Prayer was my rock.

There were so many ups and downs, so many questions, so many decisions. When Hayley first got the diagnosis, we had to absorb it all, and we had to determine if CHOP was the best place for her. What about Sloan Kettering, Mayo Clinic, Johns Hopkins, Columbia Presbyterian? It was easy to feel overwhelmed. That was the only thing that was easy. We did our research, gathering records and tests and meeting with other doctors at other hospitals and we determined that we were indeed at the right place at CHOP.

For her high-risk pineoblastoma, we followed the medical team's advice to use the St. Jude's SJMB03 protocol, which included six weeks of radiation and proton therapy and four and a half months of inpatient high-dose chemotherapy. The journey was just beginning. To prepare her for the protocol, she had to have a procedure so that her ovaries could be repositioned out of the way of radiation. They were surgically clipped to her hipbones permanently.

As bizarre as that is to grasp, it also signified that the doctors believed she would be around in adulthood.

Under the protocol, her treatment required harvesting of her stem cells before her start of six weeks of daily (Monday through Friday) cranial/spinal radiation including proton therapy. Hayley left each day at 5:45 a.m. for her daily radiation treatment and usually had extra appointments at CHOP after her radiation, so she got home in the afternoon each day. Her radiation lasted until the end of April.

She then had a planned six-week break. In mid June, Hayley started a four-month high-dose/high-frequency chemotherapy process, which involved receiving inpatient chemotherapy for three weeks. After each treatment, she would receive 2 million of her stem cells that had been harvested during a rescue process.

During her "break" she still needed MRIs, EKGs, and blood tests. We stayed pretty busy during what we called the "Break of a Thousand Appointments," but the docs tried to bundle some of the approximately thirty tests that were required prior to the start of chemo. She was able to enjoy Easter and she ate a bunch of food! Getting food into Hayley remained a constant challenge.

That Mother's Day, I will always remember how I just sat on her bed for an hour and a half straight and watched her sleep. I just stared at my precious baby girl. She truly is a gift from God, I thought. I don't know what I did to deserve her.

That May she also attended the "prom" at CHOP. It is usually for inpatients, but Hayley was there so much, they included her too. She had a blast! She danced the night away.

It was also that May that we met Laura and Celeste. We had been using CarePages, the online blog service, to post updates on Hayley and to ask for love, support, and prayers. It was a way to stay connected when we were feeling very disconnected and living in a blur. We didn't realize what a blessing it would turn out to be.

We had so many people introduce us to people who had children with brain tumours, but no one with the same kind Hayley had because it's so rare.

This is what I posted on May 17, 2011: "I received a private CarePage message from a mom of a 12-year-old girl from Canada named Celeste who was diagnosed on March 8 with pineoblastoma. We have been emailing and sharing our stories. The one difference is that Celeste has a huge appetite—my dream for Hayley. Celeste will forever be in our thoughts and prayers, and I ask all of you to pray for Celeste as well as she is still in the radiation phase of her treatment, but is following the same protocol as Hayley."

Hayley and Celeste were both 12 when they got the news of their rare brain tumors and both were on the same St. Jude's protocol. Hayley had a head start so we were able to tell Celeste what to expect.

Hayley then started the chemo phase and spent three weeks inpatient each month during her high-dose chemotherapy. That's a lot of hospital time for a little girl. For anyone.

During her inpatient stays, Hayley's doctors would closely monitor her white and red blood cell counts as they would drop and eventually bottom out at zero where she would be at greatest risk for infections. These zero levels would typically last for about a week and at this time Hayley would be confined to her room and would receive regular blood and platelet transfusions.

Typically in her third week of treatment Hayley's blood levels would rise to an acceptable level and she would be able to come home to rest up for the start of her next twenty-eight-day treatment cycle.

It was our new way of life.

The simple joy of Hayley being able to sleep in her own bed at home seemed a million years ago.

Anthony was also my rock. His sense of humour kept us going. We learned that Hayley did not do well coming out of anesthesia. She would be quite cranky. Anthony joked that she was not a happy drunk and we would have to warn future suitors. Imagining a normal happy life with my little girl doing teenage and adult activities was part of our own "small blessing protocol."

We had running jokes with the medical staff. When personnel would enter her room and ask, "How are you doing?" she would reply, "I'm in the hospital, what do you think?"

When they would ask, "Any allergies?" she would deadpan, "Needles."

Undergoing five surgeries within twenty-four days is not easy. We took any blessing we could get. Hayley was able to attend a church sleepover a month after the first surgery took place. She was able to be "normal" for an evening, to be with kids, eat pizza and ice cream, and watch a movie!

To be able to go to church, something we used to take for granted, was now a precious gift. Hayley's strength and faith were a constant source of encouragement for us all. She believed that each day was one day closer to her being completely healed.

We all share the faith that one of our friends stated so well: Christian hope is not some vague wish that things will get better. It's a confidence that God is in control and will deliver what he has promised. It's a confidence that can be acted upon each and every day.

We knew that God had BIG PLANS for this brave little girl. We still don't completely understand why we were going through this ordeal, but we continue to praise, glorify, and trust Him. We never stopped praying.

Our small blessings were many. Hayley eating Grandma's pannekaken (Norwegian pancakes), ice cream treats, every pound Hayley gained, every moment that was nausea free, every good count, every prayer from our network, every smile, every laugh.

A team of twenty, yes twenty, doctors met to review Hayley's scans and records. It was determined that the protocol was going well.

Perhaps the small blessings protocol also had something to do with that result.

We were so grateful to share it all with Laura and Celeste. We could talk about counts and meds and use all the terms that were now our standard speak but which no one else understood. We understood each other.

We understand you. You are not alone. We offer our friendship to encourage you. And we send you our love.

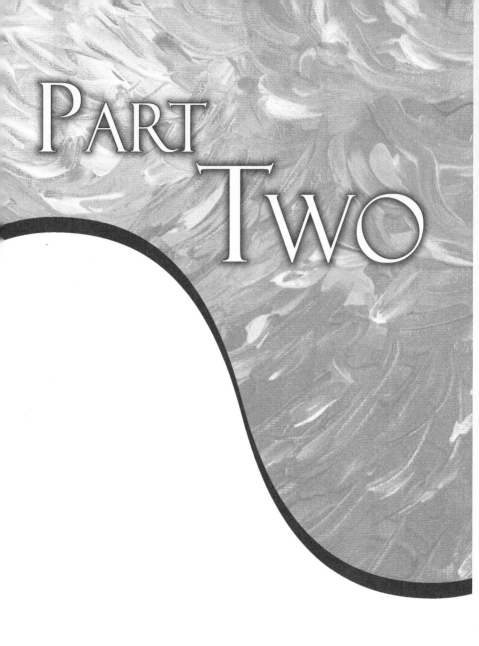

PART TWO

> *"Out of difficulties grow miracles."*
>
> JEAN DE LA BRUYERE

Chapter 4

GETTING TO KNOW ONE ANOTHER

Due to the "miracle" of the Internet, I discovered another little girl, the same age as Celeste, who was diagnosed at the same time with the same rare cancer. I reached out to her family. We connected. We were able to speak the same language and we helped each other every day. We prayed for each other, we talked and laughed and cried and celebrated and grieved together.

This is how we met.

May 15, 2011
Private message via CarePages

Hi Hayley,

My name is Laura Lane. My 12-year-old daughter Celeste was diagnosed with pineoblastoma on Mar 8 this year. She too had neurosurgery for hydrocephalus then a second surgery for a biopsy. She is receiving the same protocol and currently receiving her twenty-third of thirty-one radiation treatments before she gets a six-week break before her four to six months of chemo. I would love to connect with your family as both you girls go through this healing journey. My thoughts and prayers are with you and your family.

Sincerely,
Laura Lane

———————

May 15, 2011

Hi Laura,

My name is Laurie. My daughter, Hayley, is the person you wrote to on CarePages. We are so happy to find another 12-year-old diagnosed with the same condition. I know that sounds horrible and we are not happy your daughter is ill, but it's so hard to find anyone that is going through the same thing. We are located in New Jersey and we are currently on our break. Are you on the St. Jude's protocol? What were your daughter's symptoms? What hospital?

Laurie

———————

May 16, 2011

Hi Laurie,

Yes, I too am glad to find another family so that we can share (fill in the blank, positive and negative) our experiences. We live in Canada near Niagara Falls. Celeste had one surgery in London, Ontario, and then was transferred to Toronto Sick Kids Hospital. She is doing radiation in London but back to Toronto for chemo. We are mostly following the St. Jude protocol but with doing different parts at different hospitals, it means varying from the protocol in some areas. Celeste had headaches (two weeks) then developed double vision. Her first doctor's appointment led to the ER immediately followed by CAT scan that afternoon, then MRI by dinnertime, and emergency surgery by 9:00 p.m. That was Feb 24; she had her second surgery for a biopsy a week later and a diagnosis within another five days. She had her stem cell harvest two weeks later and started radiation Apr 11. Her last treatment is May 26.

The first week of radiation was difficult: nausea, throwing up, tired but since that week she has done terrific. Just insomnia—waking up middle of the night from the steroids. When her hair started to thin, she shaved her head and bought two wigs—one blond, one brunette— she alternates and has fun with it. Sometimes she wears hats, too! She has gained some weight with the steroids, she eats nonstop! I figure it has to be better than the alternative. She does have a "sunburn" stripe down her front and back and last week started experiencing difficulty swallowing, but since this week they are no longer radiating her spine we figure it should clear up soon.

I would love it if we could connect on the phone. I have been updating people about Celeste on Facebook but I like seeing Hayley's CarePage. Here is a link to a video I made of Celeste to help her visualize her healing. A thirty-second video can be made free if you'd like to make one for Hayley. http://tinyurl.com/l39a95t

Thank you so much for emailing me back. I hope we can be support to one another during this surreal experience.

With gratitude,
Laura Lane

———

May 17th 2011

Hi Laura,

Yes, it's been a really surreal experience. Hayley hasn't felt well for about a year. She would have episodes where her heart would race and she would turn pale and just not feel well. By the time she saw our paediatrician, she was over the episode and all of the blood tests showed nothing. I finally decided to take her to see the doctor during an episode where it was determined that she had high heart rate, high blood pressure, high calcium, low potassium, and high parathyroid. We were referred to the Children's Hospital of Philadelphia in Pennsylvania. We are from New Jersey—about one and a half hours from Philly. Our nephrologist gave her blood pressure and heart rate meds and finally stabilized her. He then ordered many CT scans, MRI scans, MIBG scans, ultra sounds, urine and blood tests, etc. He thought she had kidney issues and then changed his mind that she had tumours on her adrenals. We then went to an endocrinologist at CHOP. He said she had a syndrome called MEN2A, which would require the removal of both adrenals and her thyroid because her thyroid would become cancerous if it wasn't already. Those tests proved incorrect. He then thought she had a benign genetic condition regarding her adrenals and calcium, which also proved false. Then he thought she had parathyroid disease. At that point she began to have severe insomnia—sleeping fifteen to twenty minutes per night for eight nights with hallucinations—really crazy for hours. We brought her to the emergency room after the doctors just told us to help her sleep. She was admitted for a week and was basically told by psychiatrists to stop being a baby and to go to sleep and eat so she wouldn't be so skinny. I lost it and started screaming that of course she has anxiety. She's ill and they were telling her that she should just grow up. They placed a feeding tube in her because she was 12 years old and five feet tall and weighed only 66 pounds. After a week in the hospital, they sent her home to go to school even though she had double vision that they said was related to anxiety. I said that she was too weak, but they insisted and I started to question whether I was maybe crazy. After she attended two classes at school, I picked her up and took her to another paediatrician because I knew this wasn't right. By this time, her left eye had started to turn in. The new paediatrician said to get in the car and never let anyone tell me that double vision is only anxiety and to go straight to the emergency room. Within an hour, she was diagnosed with a tumour on her pineal gland and admitted to ICU. They performed surgery the next day to relieve the hydrocephalus. Two days later, she had a six-hour surgery for biopsy. They were not able to remove the entire tumour. Three days later, we were told that she had malignant pineoblastoma. She then had her ovaries repositioned out of the way of radiation as well as a spinal tap and bone marrow extraction. Her tumour had drop metastasized to her spine with ten to fifteen drops that had formed. We went to Johns Hopkins in Maryland for a second opinion because I was so angry that it took so long at CHOP, but he assured us that St. Jude's protocol had to be followed strictly and whether we were at Maryland, Tennessee, or Philadelphia, she would have the same treatment.

She then found out that there were no tumour cells in the bone marrow or spinal fluid. Thank God. She then had her stem cells harvested and same thing—she only needed the one day and got 11.6 million stem cells. She's gained about 12 pounds now and is up to 78 pounds. She has absolutely no appetite at all, but is getting fed through the feeding tube at night. She had six weeks and one day of radiation to the spine and brain. Two of those weeks included proton therapy, which is supposedly more gentle to the body because it targets the actual tumour instead of the whole brain and spine. She has a thick coating in her spine that they are hoping is just inflammation, but could be packed in tumour. She lost her hair, but she has a fabulous attitude—better than us at times. We have a very strong faith in God and know that he is watching over her. We know that this is such a rare tumour and you are the first person who has the same kind. We have met medulloblastoma patients, but no pineoblastoma patients. She is on break now and trying to rest as much as possible. We will be admitted for chemo on June 6. We are so thankful to God to have met you. What kind of steroids is she being given and why? Please let Celeste know that Hayley and I will be praying for her always. Yes, we definitely need to stay in touch.

Laurie

———

May 19, 2011

Hi Laurie,

I'm sorry that Hayley's journey has been such a long and confusing one. We were told Celeste's steroids are to help alleviate swelling from the radiation treatments. Celeste now has the telltale sunburn down her back.

Her father and I are divorced and last summer she went to live with him in London. So I haven't seen her since last Friday. It is a two-hour drive there so I only attend her Friday treatments. It's hard to drive four hours for a half-hour appointment every day. I will see her tomorrow morning, and then she and her 11-year-old brother and 15-year-old sister will come home for the weekend. When she has chemo, I will stay with her in Toronto Monday through Friday and her dad will be there on weekends.

I am hoping she will be officially moving back home with me, my husband, Matt, and her other brother Grayson at the end of the school year (just before chemo). She needs her Mummy! It's been hard not being able to be there for her every day through the treatments. Her stepmom takes her to the daily treatments and I travel to all the appointments and Friday treatments.

I do a lot of reading, praying and visualizing for her. I have been learning about visualization techniques and the importance of being specific in requests when we pray. I was recommended a number of books: *Getting Well Again* by Dr. Carl Simonton MD, Stephanie Matthews-Simonton, and James Creighton (how to visualize the tumours shrinking); *Anticancer* by David Servan-Schreiber (about diet); *The Healing Codes* by Dr. Alexander Lloyd and Dr. Ben Johnson MD. I have a list of other books as well. If you would like to know more, I can share more.

I will keep Hayley in my prayers as well. I told Celeste about Hayley. She is happy to meet someone who understands what she is experiencing. Perhaps they could talk over the phone or through Skype. It's getting late here and I have to put my son to bed. I look forward to your emails. Thank again

With gratitude,
Laura Lane

———

May 20, 2011

Hi Laura,

I can't even imagine what you are going through by not seeing her every day. It must be so hard on you. Hopefully her stepmom and her dad are taking good care of her. You seem to have a great head on your shoulders. I will pray that Celeste moves back home with you soon. I know that girls really need their mommies, and you need her too. It's so strange that you have a girl, boy, girl with your ex. I have a 16-year-old daughter, a 15-year-old son, and my 12-year-old daughter. In addition, our names are so similar, Laura and Laurie. It's strange that they are both 12 and both girls going through the same thing. I believe that God put us in touch with each other. I told Hayley about Celeste as well, and she would love to talk to her. How big was Celeste's tumour? Hayley's isn't large—1.5 centimetres in diameter—but her spine is the issue, ten to fifteen small drop metastases tumours as well as the fondant coating that may or may not be tumour. Thank you for the books that you recommended. I will definitely look for them. Have a wonderful weekend.

Laurie

May 30, 2011

Hi Laurie,

Today is the day I have the conversation with Celeste's dad about her moving back home with me. Please pray his heart is softened and he will simply agree that she needs to come home to me.

I posted lots of support from my friends to Hayley's CarePage. I will keep sharing the messages as they come in. We are surrounding Hayley in love and healing! I have sent out a worldwide request for prayers for her. I hope you will share this with her so that with each prayer she will get a little stronger and stronger and stronger! Someone suggested choosing a day and time to have everyone pray for both girls. I did this for Celeste two days before her stem cell harvest. It worked wonders. Maybe Tuesday at 9:00 p.m. EST would work—day before Hayley's MRI. If that works for you I will put a specific request.

If you have time today I would love to call you. Do you have Skype? Will the hospital have Internet access for Hayley while she is there? We could connect her and Celeste on Skype. Celeste will be home this weekend with me so the girls could talk if you will have time. I know this will be such a busy week for you.

With love and support,
Laura Lane

————————

May 30, 2011

Hi Laura,

I sent out the request to our churches for the Tuesday at 9:00 prayer time. It sounds great. We are leaving tomorrow at 7:00 a.m. for the hospital to begin all of her appointments prior to her admission on Monday, June 6. We are all praying hard here about your conversation with Celeste's dad. Honestly, no one here can imagine a dad not understanding how much Celeste needs you right now. I hope and pray her stepmom is loving and supporting, but I can't imagine Celeste feeling comfortable without you.

Oh, I pray so hard for you, Laura. This has been a nightmare for both of us—not to mention the girls. How is she feeling? Hayley is so tired.

Laurie

May 31, 2011

Hi Laura,

Thanks for all of the messages. They were great to hear today. I've been praying all day for you, and I hope you and your ex reached the right agreement for Celeste. We were also praying hard at 9:00 a.m. So many people have been leaving me voice mails that they are praying for you and for Celeste. I got text messages and home messages all day. We just got home, and it definitely is working. All good news about Hayley—not to mention that she's feeling much better.

With love,
Laurie

June 3, 2011

Laura,

I'm still in CHOP, and it's 6:30 p.m. on Friday. I'm sorry that I haven't been able to call you. It's been absolutely crazy here between Hayley and her tests and my mother-in-law, who also has cancer. We've been running like crazy. We are home most of the weekend. I have your numbers.

I hope to God everything went well with your meeting with your ex. How is Celeste? By the way, is it in Celeste's spine? How big is her tumour in her head? Hayley's is 1 centimeter in diameter in her head, but it is in her spine as well.

Laurie

June 4, 2011

Hi Laurie.

Celeste's birthday is on Wednesday so I am taking her and two friends for mini pedicures and manicures. Things didn't go so well on Monday. Please keep praying that her father's heart is softened and he will simply consent to her moving home with me. Celeste has been doing well since radiation ended. She has her MRI scheduled for June 20, and then her central line is being put in June 22 and the LP is June 28.

Her main tumour is 3 1/2 centimeters; she also has metastasis in her brain stem and spinal cord. It was the main tumor that blocked the flow of her brain fluid and caused the hydrocephalous.

How did Hayley's MRI go today? Celeste hasn't needed meds to stay still—she just lies there perfectly still, unless she has to go pee then she starts to squirm but who wouldn't when your bladder is full. Sometimes they let Celeste listen to music during the MRIs and she had a CD to listen to during radiation every day as well. My thoughts and prayers are with you while you prepare for Monday. Hope to talk to you soon.

Laura

While it is true that most people respect strength they don't always associate it with gentleness. But it is always from strength that gentleness arises. It is always from strength that we learn not to condemn weakness or fear or anger. Strength encourages us to empathize, to be more adaptable and make allowances. If we really wish to bring someone into our hearts and minds, a little gentleness is a powerful attraction.

LEO BUSCAGLIA

Chapter 5

A FRIENDSHIP BLOSSOMS

June 19, 2011

Hi Laurie,

Here is the link to my book I have been working on during this time. Hayley will be one of the first people to have a copy. http://tinyurl.com/kmdffyx. I am so glad to hear how well Hayley is doing. She is in my thoughts and prayers. Celeste has her MRI tomorrow morning at 7:30 a.m.—we're going to stay overnight in London tonight so we don't have to leave at 5: a.m. All my love to you and your family.

Laura

_____

June 19, 2011

Laura,

Thank you so very much!

We will keep Celeste in our prayers for a perfect MRI. We know that God is watching over Hay and Celeste, and we truly believe that she will receive good results tomorrow. Please let her know that Hay prays several times a day for Celeste!!

Love,
Laurie

_____

July 5, 2011

Hi Laura,

Hayley just told me that you needed our address.

She mentioned that you wanted to send us something. That's so sweet of you. We would love your address too. Hayley has been wanting to send something to Celeste as well.

We are really praying hard for these two brave girls and know that they will do just great. Hayley wanted Celeste to know that the first day is the worst. She threw up and was pretty tired, but felt that each day after that got easier. She thinks Celeste is braver than she is, so she feels that they will both be cured and will be able to meet and spend some time together when they are both healed.

We have been having people contact us who have been through similar situations. I always mention Celeste's name too. They've said that if you would like them to contact you for advice, moral support, etc., to please let me know. It's really difficult when people with not great outcomes contact me. It's so upsetting, but when you hear from someone with good news, it's so uplifting. Please know that we are always thinking of you.

Love,
Laurie

———

July 8, 2011

Hi Laura,

Just checking in to see how Celeste made out yesterday. Definitely ask about that chlorhexidine gluconate 0.12 percent oral rinse. One mom told us that her daughter's mouth sores were so bad that it looked like ground up beef. We will continue to pray for you guys! We need to run because we're getting another round of the chemo.

These girls are amazing and since they trust in God, they will do great!! We hope your day goes well! Back to chemo . . .

Love and prayers,
Laurie

————

July 8, 2011

Thanks Laurie,

Celeste arrived at hospital 3: p.m. yesterday, and they started her on the IV just to hydrate and co-trimoxazole to protect her lungs. The actual chemo—vincristine and cisplatin—start today about 1 p.m. They are currently adding the mannitol for her kidneys. She's had an easy evening/night and morning. We'll keep you posted as the day/evening continues.

My prayers are with Hayley today. May she have the strength she needs. The scriptures talk about taking the Lord's yoke upon you.

Matthew 11:29: "Take my yoke upon you, and learn of me; for I am meek and lowly in heart: and ye shall find rest unto your souls." (KJV)

When oxen are yoked together to pull a heavy load, they share the weight between themselves but when the Lord asks us to yoke ourselves to him he will not only share the weight of our load but will make it seem easy to bear. I know I have felt the Lord ease my burdens many times so that amazingly there was no longer any difficulty in facing the challenge.

We are praying that both girls are able to easily accept the chemotherapy with few to no side effects and that their tumours will continue to shrink and disappear. Thanks for everything, Laurie, for all your advice, prayers etc., you are sharing with us. With much gratitude for your friendship, support, and prayers.

Laura Lane

———————

July 10, 2011

Posted on Hayley's CarePages:

Thank you, God! Hayley's fever is down and she doesn't have an ear infection. Her ear situation is from the swelling in her tubes from radiation. At times during chemo, they get swollen again. Thank you, God, that the cultures are still not growing, and that the docs think she does not have an infection and that it is just one of those unexplained side effects from chemo that comes and goes. She's still very tired and her tummy hurts from the antibiotics, but in general she's doing well.

She was so happy that Grandma and Grandpa brought Taylor in for a quick visit. She missed her so much and loved hearing the stories from Taylor and Brooke's counselling days for the junior kids at Tuscarora (Christian camp in Mt. Bethel, Pennsylvania). The port issue still is not resolved. The plan is to try one more time and then put TPA in the line to see if it busts up and clots. If this doesn't work, they will probably run some type of dye test tomorrow to ensure this doesn't happen again and to see if there is a blockage.

I'm hoping we both get a good night of sleep tonight. I'm pretty tired, so I can only imagine how she is feeling between the lack of sleep and the crazy meds and feeling lousy.

Thank you for all of the prayers. We really needed them and they are working. Tomorrow we will receive 2,000,000 of her stem cells. We don't know when because they are coming from an off-site storage facility and need to be thawed out. We pray that the cells are fresh and begin working immediately. We also pray that she has no fever tomorrow and that the port kicks in and starts working as it should.

Laurie

July 10, 2011

Hi Laurie,

I was able to contact Bishop McBride from Philadelphia to arrange for a blessing for Hayley. Either he or the missionaries will come to the hospital. Either way they can give her a blessing of healing and comfort. I have been reading your posts about Hayley. So glad to hear the fever is going down. Celeste has been throwing up lots, but she has been sleeping quite well for the last few hours. We had her up for a bath to clean her up after one episode and she has been sleeping soundly since, except for her two-hour pee breaks. She has had diarrhea as well but the results haven't come back yet on whether it's from a virus or not. Her counts have been good

Friday, WBC 6.5, Poly 4.98, Hgb 109, Plat 212; Saturday, WBC 6.6, Poly 5.3, Hgb 115, Plat 225; Sunday, WBC 5.1, Hgb 106, Plat 188.

I wanted to share with you the posts I make to Facebook and the fact that people are praying for Hayley as well as Celeste:

Celeste's first day yesterday was super easy; she had a tour of the ward and settled into her room. Only treatment was some fluids to hydrate. Her stepmom, Michelle, stayed the night with her and today has been a great day for Celeste. Treatments began at 1:00 p.m. today. She has taken it so well. She has been eating and drinking well and watching TV most of the day. We are so thankful for everyone's prayers and support. Please keep praying for Hayley, the little girl from New Jersey; she has just begun her second round of chemo.

Laura Lane

July 10, 2011

Hi Laura,

We are hoping and praying that Celeste is doing well. Hayley is finally doing better. They feel that sometimes it just happens and is not because of an infection. Tomorrow is the stem cell rescue. She just took a shower. We're having port issues, so hopefully it will be resolved soon.

Thank you so much for sending the two elders to the hospital to pray for Hayley and give her a blessing. They were very nice and compassionate.

Hope all is well.

Laurie

———

July 13, 2011

Posted to Hayley's CarePages:

Hayley got a wonderful surprise from Daddy last night. He slept over the hospital with us! They stayed up and watched videos from the plays she has been in throughout the years that were directed by Louis and Stephen. She sang songs from *Joseph and the Amazing Technicolor Dreamcoat, A Christmas Carol, Honk Jr.*, etc. It was tons of fun watching her remember her parts and songs as well as everyone else's parts.

She is asked each morning to give her pain level on a scale of 1 to 10. Today, it was a zero!! The taste is out of her mouth, and the smell in the room is going away too. The docs said it smelled like coconut in here, but then we realized that it was just my shampoo. We are now having private tutoring lessons for math here at CHOP. The docs always come to our room first on their rounds because she is always up nice and early, she is cheery, eats breakfast early, brushes her teeth and does her mouthwash, changes her sheets, and uses her special body wipes all before 8:00 a.m. The docs say that most cancer patients sleep in late and that they have to wake them up for their visit—not Hayley!!

Hayley's counts surprisingly went up today. We had expected them to drop, but she received her first GCSF shot that may have boosted them a little. With this change, we expect to be at zero on the same exact day as last month. Basically, we are on a similar schedule except for the fever a couple of days ago that turned out to be basically nothing. It's nice to be able to say that so far she's handling things as expected. We ask today that Hayley is calm during the insertion of the NG tube and that she tolerates her new formula. We also ask for continued healing for Hay. Please also pray for Alexandra, Mackenzie (who is back at CHOP), Gabby, Trey, Grandma F., Mimma, and, of course, Celeste!!!

Laurie

July 14, 2011

Hi Laurie,

Glad to hear Hayley is doing well. Same for Celeste. She has an appetite back again and has been playing on the computer and doing Sudoku puzzles. I've had some frustration with watching her suffer with canker sores. No one else seems interested in encouraging her to rinse. They just want to prescribe morphine and seem to think it inevitable. Just keep giving her more and more drugs. But thankfully her temperature has been good and she's back to her normal self. Tuesday's counts were WBC 2.7, Hgb 107, and Plat 166 and Wednesday's were WBC 2.0, Hgb 103, Plat 134.

Yesterday they started the filgrastim—the G-CSF—so I'm curious about her counts today. I'd like to know if it's possible for a patient to not zero out (to hit a low of 1.0 or 1.5 or 2.0 then start climbing up again, without ever dropping down past 0.5).

I'm sure the doctors say it's impossible, but I believe in the impossible and see the impossible happen all the time! I think if we suggested to patients that things were possible we would see it happen more often. Doctors believed it was impossible for man to run faster than a four-minute mile, but after the first person did it others knew it could be done and started doing it as well. You just have to tell yourself you can. Children's minds are so open to suggestion; they will believe anything we suggest to them (that's why they believe in Santa). We should be suggesting positive healing thoughts to them instead of suggesting all the things that could go wrong.

Sorry about my rant. I wish the doctors would learn more about the importance to positive thoughts and prayer. Anyway, have a great day. I'll be back at the hospital in a few hours. If Hayley has her computer on later we can get the girls on Skype finally!

TTYS.

Love,
Laura Lane

———

July 14, 2011

Hi Laura,

I'm so sorry to hear that Celeste has the mouth sores. Are you able to suggest the chlorhexidine gluconate 0.12 percent oral rinse? I wish there was some way I could mail you a bottle, but they won't give me any extras. I offered to pay for it so we could send you a bottle, but they said it is a prescription and can't do it. If we figure something out, we will let you know. It has been amazing and she's avoided all of those sores. I totally understand what you are saying about the lack of positive healing in the hospitals. I totally agree. It's so important to think positive thoughts and to really feel the positive thoughts in order to heal. Doctors get so into the biology of things that they lose their human side.

My husband made a chart of Hayley's counts last month and put them next to this month's counts. They are very close. Today's counts were exactly the same count as last month on the same day. Our doctors screwed up the cognitive portion that should have been done during her break, so we had to do three hours today (which was a surprise to everyone including the nurses) and we have to do three more hours tomorrow.

By the way, Hayley sent a package for Celeste. It should be coming to your house soon.

Hayley just got back from all of the tests and just checked to see if Celeste was on Skype, but she's not. She said to tell you she will check again soon.

Give Celeste a big hug for us and tell her that we think she's doing amazing. We really are so lucky to have such strong girls!

Love,
Laurie and Hayley

———————

July 14, 2011

Hi Laurie,

Apparently, Celeste's mouth is getting better already. She has been rinsing with sodium bicarbonate. I have asked the doctors about the chlorhexidine, but they are reluctant to prescribe it. They said they use it with other children who move to this floor from other floors but they wouldn't prescribe it unless I insist. Unfortunately her dad and stepmom don't see the need either. They and the doctors seem to see it as inevitable that she's going to get the sores and just keep giving her morphine to deal with it. The great news is Celeste's counts went up after the G-CSF: WBC 8.7, Poly 8.5, and yesterday her WBC was 2. These numbers are higher than last week, when she arrived. Did Hayley have a similar effect when she received the G-CSF? Did her counts go up slightly? The doctors seem to think it will drop back down again and still bottom out, but I have hope that if she continues to receive the filgrastim daily that it may drop a bit down to a normal level but won't necessarily drop down to zero. I believe in amazing the doctors! I know all the prayers our girls have received are most certainly making a difference! I'm glad Hayley is feeling great as well!

Love,
Laura

———

July 14, 2011

Hi Laura,

Yes, Hayley's levels went up, too, on the first day of the G-CSF. Then they dropped. I asked also about the zero level. They said it definitely goes to zero, but I think that they don't know everything. I need to run, but we can talk tomorrow.

Laurie

July 15, 2011

Hi Laura,

One of our prayer groups wanted you to have the words
to Laura Story's song, "Blessings"

(Visit Laura Story's website learn about her music http://
laurastorymusic.com)

July 15, 2011

Hi Laurie,

That was really nice. Thanks.

Let me know what you think of "I Am the Wind"! http://
tinyurl.com/kmdffyx

With gratitude,
Laura Lane

July 17, 2011

Hayley and I keep reading your book. It's so calm
and peaceful. She actually fell asleep to it. Thanks so
much!! You are very talented. I can't wait to read your

Celeste and Hayley book. Was "I Am the Wind" your first book?

How's Celeste today? I don't have Facebook! Hayley's much better today. I really think it was the formula for the NG tube that was making her feel lousy. We have vincristine today. Hay should be fine. That one doesn't bother her too much. They are doing a urinalysis today. She doesn't seem to want to drink and her urine is very concentrated.

Laurie

————————

July 19, 2011

Hi Laurie,

I'm so glad you and Hayley like the book. How did things go with the vincristine? I was home over the weekend, and while I was gone from the hospital Celeste threw up twice Saturday and twice Sunday. I was back at the hospital Sunday night. She slept a lot all weekend and Monday she threw up again in the morning.

Her throat is really sore from the mucositis. It's affecting her throat only instead of her mouth, so they have been giving her morphine to deal with the pain, but then that makes her nauseated and she throws up which then makes her throat even more sore. Such a nasty cycle.

I spoke to a chaplain at the hospital who also is a therapeutic touch (TT) practitioner, and she is going to work
with Celeste starting Wednesday. I trained as a TT practitioner twelve years ago. TT is very effective at reducing
pain and helping patients relax, helping them heal themselves. It is a very relaxing and calming experience. If you
are interested in learning more I can track down which
nurses at CHOP do TT, and they can tell you and Hayley
more about it.

I just got back to the hospital again now after being gone
twenty-four hours and found out she spiked a fever last
night about 8:00 p.m. She has infections in both her
Hickman lines, so they are giving her three antibiotics.
Just now her fever just spiked even higher. Her counts are
quite low—WBC <0.1, Hgb 66, and Plat 30—so they
are giving her blood and platelets.

Please keep us in your prayers. I know she is surrounded
with love and prayers and she will do just fine. Thankfully
she doesn't seem much too bothered by anything. She just
says she's tired and then goes back to sleep. I keep telling
her that the more she sleeps the more and faster her body
heals. I am looking forward to Celeste feeling better soon.

I cooked up a storm for her, making lasagne rollups and
banana apple chocolate chip muffins. I froze the lasagne
in individual portions (some for Matt and Grayson, too),
so we can just heat up a portion when she wants it. I am
so thankful to have you as a friend who understands everything we are going through. All our love and prayers
to you and Hayley and your family.

With gratitude,
Laura Lane

————————

July 19, 2011

Hi Laura,

I am so sorry that Celeste is having such a tough time. That mucositis is tough. I keep hearing about it. Personally, I think Hayley has a bit of it too in her throat, but they say it looks fine and that it is just from throwing up those couple of times. She is trying now to not only use the mouthwash for her mouth, but she is also trying to gargle as far down as possible. She said it feels better today. Throwing up makes things so much worse for them. Luckily she is on easier feeds with her feeding tube and hasn't thrown up in a couple of days.

I agree with you completely on the sleep thing. I keep trying to get Hayley to nap. Yesterday she napped in the afternoon and felt so much better. Hayley's ANC is zero, WBC is 0.1, HGB is 8.8, and platelets are 35. She got platelets this morning too. The fevers are so scary. I keep hearing horror stories about kids who get fevers and infections during chemo. Some of the kids here have actually gotten 105-degree (Fahrenheit) fevers.

I honestly don't know how you do it when you can't be there all the time. I hope that your ex and his new wife are loving and that you at least trust them completely with Celeste.

I am so thankful to have you and Celeste in our lives. There are so many people praying for our girls. I am constantly getting text messages and emails that people are praying hard for the "dynamic duo" as they are called here. Even her doctors and nurses are interested in Celeste. We give them updates as well. We will keep you in our prayers always.

Hayley has been really down lately. The little girl she met in the PICU in February is no longer here. We've been trying to reach them. The parents stopped down to see me on Saturday, but I got pulled by the nurses for some questions, so they had to leave. We went upstairs yesterday (my hubby, Anthony, and I) to visit them and the room was empty. No one would tell us, out of privacy issues, what happened. I don't know if something happened or if they took her home. Supposedly the doctors said there is not much more they can do. Hayley keeps asking if we can try to find out what is going on. They are not answering phones, so please keep the family in your prayers as well.

Praying hard for the dynamic duo (Batman and Robin)!

Love,
Laurie

July 23, 2011

Hi Laurie,

I am so happy to hear about Hayley today! That's awesome! Yesterday I finally found out that ANC is the same as the Poly or neutrophils counts but our 1 = your 1,000 so Celeste's count of 0.48 is equal to 480! That was her count yesterday. She is doing much better and they have taken her off two of the antibiotics, which should help with the throwing up—we realized every time she had the Cipro she would throw up. Her bacterial infection isn't a bad one, so now she is just on one antibiotic. Hopefully it will start to clear up the diarrhea as well. That is the only thing keeping her in isolation now. Her counts are high enough so they aren't worried about her getting anything, but they are more worried until they know why she has the diarrhea. They want to ensure that she won't give a virus to someone else. Hopefully some lab results will come back to eliminate that possibility.

I came home last night and we went to the post office to collect the parcel. I had to show ID so Matt couldn't pick it up for me. We were so surprised—that box is huge! I can't wait to show Celeste! That was so kind of Hayley to send such a wonderful gift! Hayley is an amazing young woman! She has such an amazing attitude. I am looking forward to Celeste feeling better and back to her perky self again. I just got word that Celeste is moving out of isolation today! Yeah! I think she is now in a step down room. Have a wonderful weekend Laurie!

Love,
Laura

July 23, 2011

Oh Laura,

These girls never cease to amaze me. I truly believe they are both going to be fine. We will be able to somewhat laugh and give God thanks for everything someday. He is good!! He loves these girls and will heal them.

Hope Celeste enjoys her box of goodies from Hayley. Tell her we will NEVER stop praying for you.

I am so thankful to have you as a friend.

Love,
Laurie

> *"Courage starts with showing up and letting ourselves be seen."*
>
> BRENÉ BROWN

Chapter 6

SUPPORTING EACH OTHER

Aug 8, 2011

Hi Laurie,

I am so happy that you guys had such a wonderful vacation! Celeste had a great week last week. Sunday she had her picture taken with Boston Bruin Tyler Seguin and the Stanley Cup, and then Monday we were able to reserve a movie theater for a private viewing of the *Winnie the Pooh* movie. On Sunday we brought her siblings into Toronto to visit then stayed at Ronald McDonald House overnight and went to the movie together.

Celeste had her central line removed Wednesday and a new line put in on Friday. In between, we were able to take her over to Ronald McDonald House to soak in the bigger bathtub and have a picnic lunch in our room with my parents. Saturday was her first day for round two (actually day minus four) with the vincristine and cisplatin. With both rounds she has done well on this day. She even had my husband, Matt; her brother Grayson; and her aunt Steph visit. Yesterday—her day minus three with the cyclophosphamide—was much harder on her. She threw up nine times. Last night she spiked a fever but it's going down now.

Today we are doing better. She has only thrown up twice so far but she is just getting her cyclophosphamide now. Tell Hayley that Celeste commiserates with her about the throwing up. No fun. I am encouraging Celeste to sleep as much as possible. I have been working on contacting people who might cheer Celeste up. I am going to see if I can contact Miranda Cosgrove from *iCarly* to see if she could email or call Celeste as a surprise. Does Hayley like *iCarly* as well? If so I could ask her to contact Hayley as well.

Tonight when I have a better Internet access at Ronald McDonald House I plan on finishing the video for Hayley. I have been at the hospital since Friday noon without a break yet. Hopefully Celeste's stepmom will be arriving in the next hour or two so I can go have a rest.

I was sent this scripture and I thought you might like it, too.

"I will go before your face. I will be on your right hand and on your left, and my Spirit shall be in your heart, and mine angels round about you, to bear you up." Doctrine & Covenants 84:88.

All my love to you, Hayley, and your family. (Lots of our friends have Hayley in their prayers as she starts round three.)

Laura Lane

———————

Aug 8, 2011

Hi Laura,

We have been thinking of you and Celeste constantly. We mailed you another package. You should receive it soon. When you get it, just don't mention it to the doctors or nurses because they might not be happy about it.

I'm so glad that she got a new line. Hayley is throwing up quite a bit today. Actually it's more like dry heaves because she doesn't have much left in her. She does great with vincristine, but the amifostine and cisplatin really get to her. She does fine on the cyclophosphamide. It's strange how it affects people differently.

Hayley actually met Miranda Cosgrove. She came to the hospital just before we left, so Hayley was able to get a picture with her. She was really sweet. I hope you can get in touch with her.

Thanks for the scriptures. I've been reading some of the other CarePages here at CHOP and at St. Jude's Hospital. The scriptures really help to calm us and keep us positive. I think it's great that our girls really know that He is in control. Even our doctor talked to Hay about faith playing a big part. He said that he relies on what he learned in med school, his experience throughout the years, and especially his faith to guide him into helping kids get healed.

That's great that Celeste was able to get over to the Ronald McDonald House and spend time with your family. Hayley feels so much better now that she got to spend time with our family. She keeps telling everyone that she can't wait to meet Celeste when both girls are healed. We were supposed to get admitted last Thursday, but her doctor was going to be away and wanted her to wait until Monday, especially since she was enjoying herself so much. Now we're trying to get the other kids ready for school. When do your kids start school? We start around the sixth or seventh of September. I'm not even sure of the exact date. I guess I should check the calendar. I think we're good now on sneakers and school supplies.

Hayley's not feeling so well, so I better run. Talk to you later.

Love and prayers,
Laurie

Aug 14, 2011

Hi Laura,

We just wanted to check in to see how you and Celeste are doing. You are in our constant thoughts and prayers. We pray that Celeste is doing well on her G-CSF shots, and that she is not having any more fevers or central line issues. We talk about Hayley and Celeste to the doctors and nurses here at CHOP. The nurses feel that they know Celeste. Hayley is doing very well. Her counts are good, and we are just playing the waiting game, and I'm sure you are doing the same. A mom of a son with pineoblastoma contacted me a couple of months ago. Actually, he was diagnosed in January 2009 and is doing pretty well. He has something now called hypopituitarism. They thought he had thyroid issues, but it turned out to be this, which is a direct result of the tumour. I doubt our girls will get it down the road, but I think it's good for us to know of any potential side effects in the long term. Just checking to see if you received our package yet?

When Celeste is up for a Skype call, just let us know. As hard as this has been on both your family and our family, it's so great to see a light at the end of the tunnel, and to know that God the father is really watching out for these girls. We cannot imagine how families without faith get through this difficult time.

Love and prayers always,
Laurie

———

Aug 15, 2011

Hi Laurie,

I read your post this morning. That is exactly how I have been feeling—so tired! The weekend before last Celeste started her round two on the Saturday. Day minus four went well. They took Celeste off her antibiotics for the infection and her diarrhea finally cleared up. Day minus three on Sunday she threw up nine times, poor girl, and then that evening she had a fever again. They started the antibiotics again and, voilà, her diarrhea was back full force!

Monday, day minus two, I suggested to the doctors maybe it was the antibiotics causing the diarrhea so they opted to change to a different one and thankfully she has been clear of the diarrhea ever since. This is great news after weeks of it. Monday went well during the day, but Celeste threw up so much Monday night that she was put on extra fluids, which then caused her face and eye to swell up. Poor thing couldn't open her eye one morning. I went back to RMH on Monday night hoping to catch up on sleep but didn't fall asleep until 4:00 a.m.

Then Tuesday night was another up-every-hour-and-a-half-to-two-hours-to-pee night again. She moved into her isolation/healing room Wednesday and received her transplant. I don't think it smelled so bad this time, but I was gone again Wednesday night to RMH. I did laundry for her all afternoon and was exhausted, so after dinner I had a nap for three hours and then woke up to call Matt and brush my teeth. Wouldn't you know it I couldn't fall back to sleep all night. At 7:00 a.m. I called Matt again to say, "Good morning. I'm wide awake!" Then I finally fell asleep for two hours. I had to get up for an interview about my book and then back to the hospital. Celeste was doing great. She didn't throw up for days!

Sick Kids announced a talent show, so my dad brought Celeste a keyboard so she could be in the show. They brought someone to her room to film her playing her own composition plus a song from *Les Misérables*. Thankfully they are going to do the talent show every two weeks so she can keep practicing to prepare for the next show. This is a small miracle for us. She has been so down lately. She cries a lot late at night. She cries about her missing Pooh Bear and not being able to eat real food—everything tastes funny. All she ate for two weeks was watermelon because it's the only thing that tastes right. On Friday I made her some plain spaghetti with butter and Parmesan cheese. She did eat that finally.

I talked with one of the nurses late Thursday night. She is getting upset about little things and clinging to her blanket. She needs an emotional release about all her worries, but she refuses to talk about it, so I encourage her to cry about the little things instead. I am hoping to get hold of an old school counselor she had, whom she liked. Maybe she will talk to him again and pour out all the things that are worrying her.

The whole issue of where she will go when she is released from hospital is still unresolved.

I am so thankful that physically she is feeling better. I saw Matt and Grayson on the weekend for forty-eight hours and came back again last night. She had a tiny fever over the weekend so they started another antibiotic, which caused her to throw up when she received it. Today for rounds we convinced them to take her off that one. She is still on one last broad-spectrum antibiotic. She has a stuffy nose a lot but it's way better than the mucositis she had last month.

I have been asking friends to think of things that might cheer her up and help her feel like she hasn't been forgotten. I am so happy when I hear all the great support Hayley has and her great attitude. I pray I can be inspired to come up with things to help Celeste feel happier and more hopeful. I am so thankful for my own faith and knowledge that everything is going to be OK for both our girls. The peace the spirit brings is wonderful. I have always loved John 14:27: "Peace I leave with you, my peace I give unto you: not as the world giveth, give I unto you. Let not your heart be troubled, neither let it be afraid." (KJV)

I have been learning a great deal about the need to let go of our fears and truly trust the Lord. When we hold on to fear we let false beliefs (and Satan) be in control. When we trust, we give the control back to God. When we give Him the control we open up our connection to him so that he can inspire us with the actions we need to take to receive the blessings we desire. I think it comes down to believe, listen, trust, and act.

Faith is the ability to believe something enough that you are willing to act upon the belief. Do I believe God when he says everything will be OK? Do I *believe* him enough to *trust* him and am I willing to give him the control and *listen* to his prompting to *do* things that he says will make my situation better? I think about you and Hayley every day. I am so thankful for your love, support, and prayers. I can't wait until we can all meet. I know Celeste feels the same way but is just having a tough time getting excited about anything right now. This too shall pass. I will look for you on Skype. I'll ask Celeste to play a song for Hayley on Skype, maybe tomorrow night. Does she like *Les Misérables*? Celeste is practicing Cosette's song, "Castle on a Cloud." It is such a pretty song. Maybe Hayley can sing something for Celeste as well.

Love and prayers,
Laura Lane

P.S. I created an Excel program with charts/graphs to keep track of Celeste's counts. Let me know if you would like a copy to use for Hayley's counts. Oh and, no, the package hasn't arrived yet but it's always slow to get things over the border. I'll let you know as soon as it arrives. I'm very curious as to what I can't tell the doctors and nurses about!

Aug 15, 2011

Hi Laura,

Hayley is having a tougher day today. I guess it's the mucositis in her throat and esophagus. She threw up and feels better now. I'm so happy that Celeste is feeling better now. I'm sure your ex is driving you crazy. It's pretty selfish for him not to put her first. Maybe something good will come of it, and he will realize that she needs to be with you and Matt when she comes home at the end. Anthony, Hayley, and I pray for this constantly. We all agree that she needs to be with you. Anthony always tells me that children belong with their mom. God is good and will help him realize what is best for Celeste.

Hayley totally understands how Celeste feels. It's depressing for her, too, thinking about her friends enjoying the summer vacation while she is stuck in the hospital. It's totally depressing. It's depressing to me, so I can only imagine how the girls feel. They are still little girls and want to have fun and feel normal. Their faith will help them get through this time. I know they both realize that God the Father is watching over them and will heal them completely while using them to bring others to Him. He has so many big plans for these girls, but they have a right to feel down sometimes.

Anthony keeps telling me that I have to understand that between the radiation and now the chemo, it's basically putting poison into their little bodies. Of course, they will feel lousy and feel down. I think that as long as we let them know that there's nothing wrong with feeling down at times, and that they will always have us to lean on, they will both start thinking more positively. We were just thanking God that even though Hayley is feeling kind of yucky, there is a plan with the doctors to heal her. Some kids don't have that plan, and we can't imagine living like that.

Have you met a lot of families at the hospital? We tried not to, but it just happens. It's so sad when you hear some of these cases, and we can't believe how many babies have cancer. Have they talked at all about giving Celeste a feeding tube now that she's not eating much? Hayley hates it so much. She can't wait until the day when she doesn't need it. She's still so thin, but little by little, we hope she will be able to gain weight without it. Her appetite is definitely better this month than last month, but it's only enough to maintain, not gain.

Hayley loves to sing too and loves the song Celeste mentioned, "Castle on a Cloud"!

It's so funny how you mentioned that Celeste loves her Pooh Bear, etc. Hayley is exactly the same. My older daughter, Taylor, never liked stuffed animals and always tried to be more mature than her age. My son, Matthew, liked kiddie things when he was young. Hayley still loves to sleep with her pink fluffy dog named Fifi La Pinky. I wash it all the time for her to keep it clean. How are Celeste's counts? We are dropping pretty quickly now.

You are always in our thoughts and prayers,
Laurie

Aug 17, 2011

Hi Laurie,

My friend is helping me find someone in Philadelphia who can give you a sample of Kangen alkaline ionized water. It will help with Hayley's esophagus. They will try to sell you a machine but maybe you can rent one instead like I am doing. The machine takes tap water and runs it through a filter and electrolysis plates to split the water into acidic water (good for cleaning) and alkaline water (good for drinking). It is great for dealing with heartburn, acid reflux, and other similar problems. I really think it would help Hayley. You can get a free sample (gallon jug or more) to try it out. Because it is ionized (negative ORP) they call it living water. The body absorbs it better than regular tap water so it hydrates the body better, as well. It tastes better so you drink more of it, too; it seems easier to drink somehow. It helps with kidneys as well so I hope it can really help both our girls. I have a rental machine in the bathroom at Ronald McDonald House and I bring a jug of water at a time over to the hospital.

Sick Kids is really strict with a low-bacteria diet for Celeste, no restaurant or fast food whatsoever until three months after chemo ends plus a bunch of other no's. Only home-cooked or hospital-prepared food. Not even from their own cafeteria downstairs. So I am awaiting approval that I can bring the water in for Celeste. In the meantime I drink it myself.

Celeste's ANC is 20 today. It was zero yesterday, so we're heading back up again. I told Celeste if things go as well as last month or better she should be engrafted (ANC 500) by Saturday! Then she can move back to the bigger step-down room. I like how Hayley can stay in one room the whole time. Celeste can't leave this room for any reason until she engrafts. She has mucus only in her nose this month—just a bit stuffed up. She has gagged on it a few times, coughs, and then throws up, but that is much better than the pain in her throat last month. They were giving her morphine for the pain last month, which then made her nauseated and caused her to throw up. This then made her throat feel worse—yuck.

She's doing great this month in comparison. Last night she had a fever for about 10 min then after the doctor came in to say we have to put her back on the Cipro antibiotic just to be safe until the cultures comes back, they took her temp again and it was normal again. We don't like the Cipro because she gets nauseous when they give it to her and she throws up. But I'm going to ask about the cultures now to see if she can be taken off the Cipro as soon as possible.

Let me know if you will be available on Skype later and I can show you a technique to help Hayley go to sleep. I think about you guys all the time, always telling everyone about our friend Hayley from New Jersey!

Thanks for being there, Laurie; I don't think I could have made it through all this without you. I haven't really connected with any of the other parents here. I am so thankful the Lord brought us together!

Love,

Laura

————————

Aug 23

Hi Laurie,

Celeste is doing great this month / this week. No mucositis! She engrafted on Friday (ANC 530), one day sooner this month. Her ANC hit 2080 yesterday! And her WBC hit 6.9 or 6,900 today but her ANC did drop a bit to 1,730. She has a rash, which they say is common with engraftment. Not a big deal. Today she also had her kidney function test this morning and an MRI this evening at 9pm.

She has been quite grumpy all day but that's better than being sick. I would really like to see her go home for a week this month. It would be so great for her spirits. I am so happy Hayley is up singing and dancing.

Matt, Grayson, and I got away for forty-eight hours to Lee, Massachusetts, for a Dodge Power Wagon truck rally. A number of people drive up from New Jersey to attend. Thank you for the care package! It arrived just before we left. You guys are so great. I'd still like to call sometime. If we don't connect on Skype maybe I can just call through to Hayley's room.

Happy belated birthday, Laurie! We have both spent our birthdays in hospital with our girls this year. I'll let you know about the MRI as soon as I know. Praying that her tumour and cyst have shrunk and disappeared completely! Praying the same for Hayley too!

All my love,
Laura Lane

P.S. I have been having lots of the trust-fear-trust-fear-trust feelings as well this week. Wow, this is quite the learning journey we are on.

———————

Aug 23, 2011

Hi Laura,

I totally understand the trust-fear feelings. I do it all the time. Sometimes I am great and totally trusting. Other times, it's just plain scary. I want to just trust all the time, but we see what's happening around us with other kids and it's so hard.

We are praying like crazy for Celeste's MRI. We believe that you will see big changes like we did. I struggled for a long time, wondering whether we chose the right treatment for Hayley, but I really think this St. Jude's protocol will work.

I'm glad you got the package. I was afraid that it might not get through customs. We sent it while we were in North Carolina. My brother said to tell you that if you like it and need more, just tell him. The wipes are great too. They are usually used prior to surgery.

The Power Wagon truck rally was probably exactly what you, Matt, and Grayson needed. We have those grumpy days, too, and, from what I hear, a lot of people have that as well. Hayley threw up her tube last night and her tummy is really bothering her. We think we will be going home tomorrow for about a week or so. We are anxiously awaiting Celeste's MRI results. Between my phone issues here and Hayley having trouble getting onto Skype, it's been a pain in the neck this month. We hope next month is a lot better.

Love and prayers,
Laurie

———————

Aug 23, 2011

Hi Laurie,

We just found out that, if everything goes well this week, Celeste goes home Friday afternoon until September 1! I am so happy! Thank you for your prayers! We have to wait until Friday because they want to wean her off her meds and do a lumbar puncture on Friday.

When does Hayley start her last round? (That's so cool to say—last round—she's almost done!) You can see the light at the end of the tunnel! I'll email you as soon as I hear about the MRI. Actually, I'm going to go down the hall now to ask if they have the results yet. We haven't seen the doctor yet today. Celeste went back to sleep after her tests. She gets grumpy when they wake her up for tests especially if she doesn't know beforehand that it's scheduled. OK, I'll email you again soon!

Love and prayers,
Laura

Here was my Facebook post today:

Woohoo—great news! Celeste (if all goes well) gets to come home for five days! This week is lots of tests and then Friday afternoon she should be discharged until September 1! Yesterday were her kidney function test and MRI. This morning were the ECHO and EKG. This afternoon are audiology and pulmonary functions tests, and then Friday she has a lumbar puncture. We just have to keep her fluid intake up and get her eating more. She requested more watermelon for lunch and hopefully she will let me cook something for her for dinner, casserole or spaghetti. I'll make whatever she wants. I'm so happy to know she gets to come home this month! Thank you everyone for your prayers! Hayley is doing well, too, and gets to go home for a week as well! Oh, and there is another "Sick Kids Got Talent" show again on Friday so we'll get Celeste practicing again so she can play another song in the show. We are also going to arrange for her to go down to Marni's lounge on Thursday to make cookies and up to the Starlight lounge on Wednesday. She is looking forward to Bingo on Thursday, too. It's going to be a great week! Can you tell I'm excited?! I'll let everyone know about the MRI as soon as I hear anything, hopefully today!

Aug 25, 2011

Hi Laura,

Just checking to see if you got the MRI results and to see how Celeste is feeling.

Hayley is home. Her ANC is at 2,610 today! Thank you God!

Laurie

Aug 26, 2011

Hi Laurie,

Celeste just had a rough eighteen hours of throwing up and fevers. She's fine now, but it sure wasn't fun for a while there. Her MRI came back with no changes this time but because it shrank 84 percent last time. The last 16 percent can be slower to get rid of because it may be a different type of tissue left in the tumour that just takes longer to break down. We also received word that Celeste can't be discharged now until Monday when her antibiotics have finished their full course. Also they don't need to do the lumbar puncture tomorrow.

We are really thankful for that. I am so glad Hayley is home now. That's so awesome. Celeste's ANC have made it up to the 2,000s and 3,000s on Tuesday and Wednesday as well. I don't know whose house Celeste is going home to now on Monday. I hope and pray that her father will just let her come home to me, seeing as he will be working.

Celeste had a great visit with Desiree, Connlan, Grayson, and Matt yesterday before she got sick. We're hoping to do the same Sunday afternoon as well. I'm looking forward to hearing about the fun stuff Hayley gets to do while she is home.

TTYS.

Love and prayers,
Laura

———

Aug 28, 2011

Hi Laurie,

Here is the video of Hayley that I promised. I was able to come home this weekend and finish it. I hope you like it. I think it turned out beautifully!

http://tinyurl.com/nnnhjzr

Celeste's counts have been great (except her platelets) but she had another fever for a bit yesterday, so she won't be able to come home before she starts round three on Thursday.

Last week was disappointing; all the fun stuff we wanted to have had to be cancelled due to medication problems. Wednesday they tried her on a new drug for her lungs (can't remember the name now) to protect against pneumonia, but it ended up making her throw up for four or five hours and she had fever and chills, so then she was put on antibiotics, which also make her throw up. The next day, when she was finally feeling better, one of the nurses made a mistake and gave her a double dose of the antibiotics, making her throw up more needlessly. Poor thing. I know she is disappointed about not going home, so I will have to double my efforts to find ways to cheer her up. Maybe we can get a day pass one day to go out and do something fun.

How is Hayley enjoying her time at home? We're you affected by the storm at all? The storm clouds have reached all the way over to our house west of Niagara Falls, quite a ways inland. It hasn't started raining yet but it may later in the day. Take care and have a wonderful Sabbath. (Do you take Hayley to church when she is home? Or is it too risky with so many people there and risk of infection?)

Love and prayers,
Laura

Aug 29, 2011

Hi Laura,

Yes, we take Hayley to church, but it was cancelled on Sunday due to the storm. We've been out of power for a few days, but it came on about an hour ago. Thank you, God!

I'm so sorry that Celeste can't come home. We take the pneumonia meds too. We call it Bactrim. Hayley hates taking them because the pills are huge, so she has to break them in half. We will continue to pray that Celeste does much better this round. She's such a brave young lady.

Laura, that video was amazing. Everyone here is crying. Thank you so much for doing that for us. We just love it.

We will keep praying for you and Celeste as she begins round three on Thursday. We think we won't begin for another week or so. Monday, September 5, is Labor Day here (holiday), and they won't admit on the weekends. We found out that they don't like the "weekend" staff to be on when she has her first day of chemo, so our only other option is September 8 (Thursday) because Thursday, September 1, isn't 28 days and they won't start early. I know what you mean about the platelets. They are the worst with Hayley too. It seems like she always needs platelets. They loaded her up on them on the day we left to try to give her a boost, so I'm hoping tomorrow they will say she is good and doesn't need any.

I'm trying so hard to be positive, but sometimes it is so hard. I know you totally understand. There are a few parents of kids who have been on the St. Jude's protocol in the past for medulloblastoma—not exactly the same, but they said that if you want to talk, just let me know. They are all nice, but it's hard because it's not the same type of tumour. Most of the ones we have been talking to are having some later issues, thyroid issues, spine issues, drugs, hair. Hayley has what she calls a reverse mohawk— hair on the sides, but a big strip in the middle is missing. I try to stay positive that our girls can return to normal, but it's hard when you see that others are not adjusting completely. I will try to get out of this negative mindset and think positively. Thank God for our faith. How do people do this without it?

Love, peace, and prayers ALWAYS,
Laurie

———————

Sept 6, 2011

Hi Laura,

Just checking to see how Celeste is doing. You are in our constant thoughts and prayers. We are back to the hospital on Thursday, and I'm sure you've seen the horrendous things going on at CHOP with a couple of the kids on my CarePages. It's so sad, and it's so hard to stay positive.

Anyway, we hope Celeste is having a better month and we pray she will be able to go home this month. How are things going? How are you doing? Is your ex going to let Celeste come to your house?

Love,
Laurie

———————

Sept 6, 2011

Hi Laurie

Celeste is doing so well now! Her fevers stopped last week, they took her off the antibiotics so now the diarrhea is gone too. Her counts are finally better: WBC has been over 10,000 for more than six days. Her Hgb are level at 87 and platelets are finally staying up past 50. They went as low as 9 last week.

She was eating like crazy yesterday. She ate watermelon, pork chops and rice, three hard-boiled eggs, and then roast beef and mashed potatoes. Today she will be Hep-Locked (not connected to the IV) from 9:00 a.m. to 5:00 p.m., so we can have a day pass.

Now that the long weekend is over we're waiting to hear from the doctors about when round three will actually begin and maybe she can go home for a few days in the meantime! Yeah! I'm so glad to share good news with you!

Hayley and Celeste are very special girls and they are going to continue to pull through this with flying colors. Keep Trusting the Lord. I know I have continually had a peaceful feeling that everything is going to be OK. If Heavenly Father has blessed you with the same feeling then let him carry the load.

I know it's hard when other children are called home but we can find purpose and good in all things when we can see things from the Lord's perspective. There is goodness to be found and lives are still touched and changed for the good when little ones go home to Heavenly Father. My sister was 7 when she returned to him. Her passing gave me the strength to be who I am today. Every experience we have had in our lives has made us the strong women we are today.

The Lord is strengthening those families as they pass through these trials just as He does us. My thoughts and prayers are with you continually. I can't wait for the day for our families to meet in person. My dad wanted to call you sometime to say hello as well. What number can he call you at? I recall that Hayley's birthday is this month. What day? We would love to wish her a happy birthday. Don't worry Hayley is going to have an awesome month and will amaze her doctors even more. Just keep telling her that!

Love always,
Laura

———

Sept 6, 2011

Laura,

I just wanted to tell you that you are such an amazing woman and mom. I am in awe of your strength and faith. Hayley and I were just talking about how lucky we are that you and Celeste have come into our lives. We just cannot wait to meet you in person!! We pray for a good night for Celeste.

Love and hugs and prayers, of course,

Laurie

Sept 15, 2011

Hi Laurie,

Celeste had a rough night Tuesday night but hopefully will be back in her room today. Here is the posting I made on Facebook for you to read the simplified version but I'll email you again later when I have a free moment. I am so happy to hear how well Hayley is doing! It's wonderful to hear.

All my love,
Laura

Celeste did well on Monday; it's always an easy day, the first day of chemo with the vincristine. Monday night she did spike a fever, which made it a more difficult night. Tuesday she started out with some swelling from all the extra fluids they were giving her, but she didn't throw up as much this time as she did the other months with the two chemo drugs she gets. Unfortunately the fever spiked again and the swelling got worse and her blood pressure dropped so at 4:00 a.m. we had to go down to the second floor critical care unit so they could give her meds that they don't have on her floor and monitor her. Wednesday she had improved greatly. The swelling has gone down some, and they have started to wean her from the meds and her blood pressure is stabilizing. She isn't happy about being there but she should be back in her own room again, hopefully within the next twenty-four hours. It means she also didn't have to have any chemo drugs on Wednesday and today they will go ahead with the stem cell transplant a day early. Please pray that she can be comfortable with all the extra IV lines, that her blood pressure will normalize, the swelling will go down completely, and that her body can fight off whatever infections caused the fevers. She is looking forward to eating again and has requested peanut butter and jam.

Sept 15, 2011

Hi Laura,

We were just praying for Celeste and hoping things were going well. I'm so sorry that she had such a rough time. It's funny because I was just talking to my brother. He always asks about Celeste, and I told him that Celeste did so much better than Hayley during radiation and had energy, was eating, and even went to school sometimes. Hayley handled it much worse than Celeste and couldn't go to school, was exhausted, had no appetite, and was so nauseous. Chemo seems to be the other way around for them. From what I hear, you do well with either one or the other. We are so thankful to God that Celeste seems to be getting better and better and is hungry for peanut butter and jam.

We had a bit of a fiasco the other night. We had a new nurse who made a mistake and injected Hayley with someone else's medicine. She never looked at her wristband at all. Then she panicked and wouldn't tell me what she injected. I couldn't sleep all night, and finally in the morning, they determined that it was someone else's G-CSF shot, which wasn't dangerous because it was a baby's dose. The nurse can't work on the floor anymore. Hayley had a spike in her ANC from the two doses, but she's fine now.

We will keep praying for Celeste and you and for your ex to let Celeste go home to your house. My whole family is praying so hard for you. We've asked our youth pastor to pray as well.

All my love,
Laurie

———

Sept 19, 2011

Hi Laurie,

Every time you mention how depressing it is there I want to make sure I share my good news with you. Celeste is doing great! She looks so much better this week. All the cultures came back negative so they don't know why she had a problem last week, but as far as I am concerned it doesn't matter because this week everything is back to normal.

She is eating up a storm. She looks great. She's playing games and Skyping; she has her sense of humor. She watched our favorite TV show all weekend: *Doctor Who*. She's doing her physio. She doesn't have any mucositis at all this month. Her potassium was low but now it's getting better and she's eating banana milkshakes too.

I am so happy for Hayley, too! Our girls are doing great and we can celebrate their victories soon. I don't have any doubt about the tumours shrinking. How can those tiny tumours compete against the love and faith these girls are surrounded with?

I'm sorry you have to see the suffering around you, but it is making you and Hayley more compassionate. These are things you and her will never forget and are making you stronger. When Celeste was in a four-bed ICU room for an hour last week before they moved her to a private room, I could feel so many spirits watching over those children. The room was filled. (It was a bit overwhelming for me but a good reminder that those children are never alone during their fight whether they make it or not.)

Just remember how special you are to have such a special daughter and to be witness to her greatness as she amazes everyone with her faith and strength and reliance on the Lord. She chose you to be her mom and to help her through this. You are amazing too! I think we should start planning the Hayley & Celeste celebration party soon.

All my love,
Laura

P.S. We had a similar thing happen with meds: Celeste was given a double dose of antibiotics one night. One nurse had given the dose three hours early and hadn't logged it before the other nurse took over, so she was given it again. I was very upset. It didn't do any harm as far as the doctors were concerned, but the drug makes Celeste nauseated when she receives it and she throws up. It caused her needless discomfort throwing up when she shouldn't have had to. I became much more watchful about what drugs she was getting and when. They have finally stopped using that drug that makes her throw up and the other one that gives her diarrhea and switched to a different antibiotic that doesn't bother her in the same way.

———

Sept 20, 2011

Hi Laura,

Thanks for the good news about Celeste. He is truly watching over our babies. I'm so thrilled to hear that Celeste's cultures came back negative. I guess as they get beaten down, it's harder to recover, but we are so lucky to have such strong girls with such strong faith. I know that today will be a better day for Hayley. She's sleeping now, so I am happy that she's getting some extra rest.

Please know that you and Celeste are ALWAYS in our prayers. It's so sad to see all of the suffering, but we still trust and know that He is in control. I was watching a Christian show last night that said God the father expects us to completely trust him even when things seem down. I always think of Psalm 50:15: "Then call on me when you are in trouble, and I will rescue you, and you will give me glory." (NLT)

Love and hugs,
Laurie

———

Sept 21, 2011

Hi Laura,

I hope things are going well with Celeste. Hayley is feeling pretty well. Her rectum is bothering her. She has much less mucositis this month, but I think it's from hard bowel movements even though she is taking quite a few meds to soften them. Otherwise, we are just waiting for the counts to continue to rise. How are things going for Celeste?

It was so nice to talk to your father yesterday—what a kind and nice man. You are really lucky to have him as your dad and Celeste's grandfather. We talked for a while about how brave the girls are and he told me about his stay as a child in the hospital. I told him that my dad also has rheumatoid arthritis—strange that both grandfathers have it. We also talked about the girls meeting someday and how much our talks (yours and mine) have been comforting and a help.

It's been tough here lately, but I'm trying to stay positive. Sometimes it's easier said than done, but it's what God wants from us.

Hope all is going well. Give Celeste a hug for us.

Love and prayers,
Laurie

———————

Sept 21, 2011

Hi Laurie

Good news: Today was day plus six with the vincristine and Celeste had no problems whatsoever! She even called me at Ronald McDonald House at 6:00 p.m. to request roast beef, mashed potatoes, and Yorkshire pudding! I was so excited because it means not only that she didn't throw up but she has an appetite as well.

Last week they put her on steroids but started weaning her off of them since the weekend. Her blood pressure has been a little high for a couple of days this week because of the steroids, but after it's being low last week it was much easier to deal with. Her potassium was also low, so she had to take some huge pills and eat banana milkshakes and banana splits. It's better today as well.

The vincristine has affected her hand coordination a little, but an occupational therapist is helping her with that. It shouldn't take long to fix that. She is squeezing clay to work on improving her hand/finger strength and we are encouraging her to play the piano to help as well. She also has a physiotherapist working with her to improve her leg strength.

She doesn't get as much opportunity to walk around like Hayley does. Her regular room is so much smaller, and when she is in the isolation room from days zero to ten she only takes one step over to the commode and then back to her bed. Last month she had to be taught to climb stairs again because she hadn't used those muscles in two months, but then when she went home she was able to go up and down stairs (with help) to get to her room or the bathroom. It shouldn't take long for that to improve as well.

They finally got Celeste on antibiotics that don't bother her stomach. The first two months every time she was on antibiotics she kept getting diarrhea and her bum got pretty sore from that, so she knows how Hayley feels, although for the opposite reason. Celeste is doing so well this week. I suggested to her that she should engraft by Saturday, which would be the same as last month and again a day earlier than the previous month.

Hopefully she can go home for a week this time once she does all the required tests next week. Hayley is our example on this one! I need Celeste to know it's possible because the doctors don't talk about it. I keep watching the posts about Hayley's counts. She'll be done in no time.

I'll make sure everyone is praying about her upcoming MRI. My dad said he really enjoyed speaking with you as well. He looks forward to talking to Hayley sometime soon as well. Don't forget as you remain positive and keep doing all you are doing for Hayley, you are an inspiration to others.

"Let your light so shine before men, that they may see your good works, and glorify your Father which is in heaven." Matthew 5:16 (KJV)

Others need to see your example and feel the strength you receive from your faith and trust in the Lord. "Peace I leave with you, my peace I give unto you: not as the world giveth, give I unto you. Let not your heart be troubled, neither let it be afraid." John 14:27 (KJV)

Love, hugs, prayers, friendship and gratitude,
Laura

Sept 22, 2011

Laura,

I am so glad that Celeste is doing so much better. She is an amazing young woman, and I am so thrilled that she's eating so well and handled the vincristine so well. Yes, we are really lucky that we have such a big room. Hayley is able to move around quite a bit here and I really believe it has helped her tremendously. The doctor just walked in, so I'll talk to you later.

Hugs and prayers,
Laurie

Sept 22, 2011

Hi Laurie,

I told Hayley on Skype about the paintings I have been doing late at night at Ronald McDonald House when I'm not at the hospital. Last night I did these painting inspired by colours Celeste chose: blue, green, purple, and silver. I would like to do another set of paintings next week with colours that Hayley thinks would be nice. Last week I did a set at Matt's request using black, red, gold, and silver. She can choose any four colours and I will see what sort of paintings those particular colours inspire me to paint. Hope today is a good day for both girls.

Love always,
Laura

———

Sept 22, 2011

Laura,

Hayley thinks your paintings are amazing. Between your books and now your paintings, wow, you really are talented. Hayley loves purple, blue, pink, and yellow. She can't wait to see what you come up with. Hayley is doing much better today, and we pray for a peaceful, healing, and calm day for Celeste.

Love and prayers,
Hayley and Laurie

———

Sept 27, 2011

Hi Laurie,

I'm so glad we were able to talk yesterday. I'm sure it was a busy day. Thanks for taking the time. I'm so happy Hayley is home. Please give her a big hug for me. Tell her when she worries about being home that home is the BEST place to heal because it's a place filled with LOVE and happiness. Help her see HOME as a healing safe place. Now she gets to rest and heal.

Healing is something doctors can't do for us. It is something we, with God's help, do. We accept the work doctors do then allow our bodies to heal. And if she or anyone else ever wonders why she isn't out doing other things yet just have her remind people "I'm healing right now! It's the most important thing for me to do right now." Even though we can't see healing going on inside us, just remain positive and have faith that it continues to happen just as you have faith in God that his mighty hand is at work.

I painted a few paintings last night with the colours Hayley chose. I have one more that isn't done yet. I'll show it to you when it's done as well. Let me know which ones are your favorites. This morning I am going to speak to someone at the Art Gallery of Ontario about putting them in a gallery. Pray that they will love the idea of showing art that I created while at Ronald McDonald House and that I can bring awareness to people about RMH, Sick Kids Hospitals, and Hayley and Celeste. I might even sell some of the pieces as a fundraiser. I have done twenty-four paintings so far in the last three months. I'd rather paint than watch TV.

Love and hugs,
Laura

P.S. I don't remember if I told you yesterday but I actually heard the doctor and nurses say about Celeste: "She is amazing!" I knew it would happen but now I finally got to hear those words! It was one of the positive statements I had put in the video about Celeste! http://tinyurl.com/l39a95t

Sept 28, 2011

Oh Laura, they are so beautiful. She absolutely loves them. Her favorite is the third one, *Waves,* but she thinks they all are amazing. We are praying hard when you talk to the gallery. Any word yet on whether Celeste will do next month's treatment or not? She really is amazing. I really believe that their faith and determination are a big part of it. You have been such a wonderful mother to Celeste, and I'm sure more than ever that she is grateful to have you in her life. I truly believe that God will give her the courage to talk to your ex about moving in with you. She really needs your positive attitude and faith. I really believe that you are the reason that she is doing so amazingly during this treatment. You have such positive energy, and we are so amazed when we see the strength that both of you have. God has worked such wonders in your daughter and will continue to do so.

Hayley is doing well, too. I have to go to Minnesota this weekend to visit my daughter, Taylor, for parents' weekend at her school. Hayley's not too crazy about my leaving, but I need to be a mom to Taylor too. Matthew and Taylor need me. I'm sure you know what I'm talking about because you've been there so much for Celeste between traveling back and forth and staying at the hospital. They really need us, but we both have other kids that need us as well. I feel like I've given Hayley 90 percent and only 5 percent to each of the other two for so long now. I want Hayley to depend a little less on me and give them a little more. I think it will be good for all of them. I believe that

God is truly in control and will heal both of our babies, and I know you believe this too.

Love and prayers,
Laurie

———————

Sept 30, 2011

Hi Laurie,

Here's the great news: Celeste went home today. She's done! We're not doing round four!

After consulting the people running the St Jude's Protocol, Dr. Doyle learned that they don't seem to find much difference between kids who finish three rounds and those who finish four. So in order to save Celeste from getting sick again or worse this month we (and she) opted out of round four. So she headed back to London this afternoon.

It was very hard for me to see her go. We found out yesterday and I had such a hard time keeping it together. I am going to miss her terribly.

It was even more difficult when staff kept approaching me about things that needed to be arranged for home then I had to tell them that, no, she wasn't coming home with me and I would want to cry all over again.

Then nurses and other parents would say, "She's going home, that is terrific! Aren't you excited?" Then they would look at my face and I'd have to explain again and cry all over again. It just breaks my heart.

How am I supposed to accept that now I have to just stop mothering her and I can only do so from a distance again? It hurts so badly.

Thank you for all your love and support. I don't think I could have done this, gotten through the last few months without you and Hayley and your faith and hope.

Please keep praying for us. I have come to love you and your family so dearly even though we haven't met. I am so thankful that the Lord brought our families together. I will write more later, but I think a good night's rest is in order now.

All my love and gratitude,
Laura

> *"Courage isn't having the strength to go on—it is going on when you don't have strength."*

> NAPOLEON BONAPARTE

Chapter 7

THE ROAD TO RECOVERY

Oct 4, 2011

Oh Laura,

I am so happy for you that she doesn't have to endure that horrendous last round. That's so fabulous, but I am so sad for you that she is going home with your ex. I believe with all my heart that this will work itself out. You are a wonderful mother who has done everything in her power to help her daughter heal. God loves you and Celeste so much and I am 100 percent positive with the continued prayers, this will work out. We will NEVER, EVER stop praying for this as well as for Celeste's health.

We love you and Celeste so very much and are so thankful to God for bringing you into our lives. I feel in my heart that these girls will be fine and that he has big plans for them. Laura, please try to stay as focused as always and never lose faith that this will work itself out. Celeste has gotten so used to your being around and is going to miss you terribly. I know that she will be talking to your ex, and my hope and prayers are that he will see that it is best for her to be with you.

Hayley is doing well. I went to Minnesota to visit Taylor at school for parents' weekend. It was so good to see her and she's so happy being with her five cousins at a Christian school and meeting so many wonderful people.

Laura, we will always pray for you. Please stay in touch with us, too. We love you so much.

Laurie

———————

Oct 13, 2011

Hi Laurie,

Celeste had an MRI yesterday. A week last Tuesday she threw up, and then later in the evening she complained about her vision. She couldn't see to the left in her peripheral vision so Michelle took her to ER. They did a CAT scan and everything was fine. She had a follow up with a neuro-opthamologist and he thinks it may just been a type of migraine common in kids her age. But they still wanted to double check by doing an MRI. The preliminary report came back as OK and her tumor has shrunk some more! I don't know exactly how much yet but I'll let you know as soon as I have numbers.

She and her brother and sister came home for the weekend and because it was our Canadian Thanksgiving we had a three-day weekend! It was terrific to have the whole family home together. Celeste is using a cane for balance when walking around the house and she does have a walker if we go out for longer walks, so that if she needs to stop to rest she can use the built-in seat. Her appetite is quite small now that she is off the steroids and we have the same problem of saying, "Just have one more bite." Although Tuesday, at her dad's, that backfired twice in that one more bite was just too much and then she threw it all back up.

I did rest a lot our first week back—I had to rest because I came down with a cold and was determined to be better by Friday when Celeste was coming home for the weekend. I am feeling stronger and more positive again, learning to surrender to the circumstances and find the positive in it all again.

I know everything will be OK. Celeste's blood counts have risen. She hasn't needed any platelets or blood so far (knock on wood). Yesterday her platelets were 62, up from 38 and 49 previously. Her Hgb was only 82 but as long as she is feeling OK—not too tired, etc.—then they aren't going to give her a blood transfusion this week. Her WBC and ANC are 7,500 and 4,200!

I am so glad Hayley is doing equally well. I read your last CarePages post. I am glad you had your break and time to visit with your daughter. Desiree and I went out Saturday to get haircuts and ice cream, and then, after Celeste went to bed, she and I stayed up making homemade apple pie and lemon meringue pie for our Thanksgiving dinner. She thanked me for teaching her how to make pies, and the next day helped me prepare most of the turkey dinner. Celeste was able to eat a few things, but she wants a proper roast beef dinner with beef gravy next time because the turkey gravy just didn't taste right.

I also put the girls to work cleaning up their room, pulling out old stuff and clothes, and then Celeste and I went through the box of stuff Hayley had sent her. I had showed it to her in July but I guess she doesn't remember much from July because of all the drugs. So it was like it was all new again! Thank you once again. She did the Adlibs in the car for an hour on Monday and now has lots of things to keep the boredom away at her dad's house. I told her to remember that if she goes on Skype, that Hayley is home all day as well. So maybe they can email what times are good to look for each other on Skype when everyone else is a school. She naps most afternoons but maybe just before lunch or just after lunch might work on days they don't have doctor's appointments.

This weekend Matt and I are going to go up north for the weekend for a much-needed break. Do you and Anthony ever get to have a break together? I hope so. When you think you could get away for a few days, we have a special spa we like to visit. We'd love it if you came with us some time. It's a wonderful way to relax. I think about you guys all the time and love you too!

With all my love,
Laura

Oct 13, 2011

Hi Laura,

I was just thinking about you this morning and said that I needed to email you too. I'm so glad that Celeste's tumour has shrunk some more. Thank God that everything seems to be normal on her scans. We talked to a girl that went through the St. Jude's protocol a couple of years ago. She said she was nauseous and feeling really tired the first year after treatment and still feels tired. I guess we just have to be patient. Hayley is being a little lazy at times. I have a hard time getting her up to take a walk or just getting her to do much of anything. Thankfully the teachers are coming here and it forces her to do her homework.

She's getting stronger each day, but that appetite problem is such a problem. I see you are having the same issue. I usually don't like her to eat a lot of junk, but she doesn't feel like eating anything healthy. The doctors tell me to let her eat whatever she wants, but as a mom, we want them to eat healthy food. I try to sneak it in, but she fills up so quickly. She really doesn't want the feeding tube, so she tries to eat. I'm a little worried that after our blood test today (results aren't back yet) and her appointment with the doctor next week, she most likely show that she's lost some more weight. Sometimes I think that because you and I are very proactive people and very involved in our girls' lives, we are expecting too much too soon. I keep telling myself that both girls are actually doing really well.

I totally understand what you are saying about the cane and walker. We have a wheelchair for Hayley when she gets tired. I hate taking it on our walks because I feel like she doesn't push herself when she knows it is there, but I really don't want her to get overtired either. It's such a fine line to walk.

I'm so glad you got to spend time with all of your kids. We are still praying hard here for everything to work out for you. It's very hard when there is a divorce.

We haven't been able to get away really because Hayley is so afraid to be away from me. I went for almost two days to see Taylor at school, but Hayley called me continuously and ate and slept terribly. I know she needs to deal with things, but I made her a promise that I wouldn't leave her alone until she felt comfortable. I'm trying to wean her a little from me, but it's hard for her and it's hard for me after everything she went through. I don't know how you have the strength to deal with Celeste being at your ex's house. You are truly a remarkable person with a tremendous amount of faith. I really hope his new wife is kind and compassionate towards Celeste and towards you and understands how hard this is on you.

We will keep praying and thinking of you. I'll mention to Hayley about Skype.

Love,
Laurie

Oct 21, 2011

Hi Laurie,

I saw your post about Hayley platelets being up to 136 (that's so awesome!) so I told Celeste about it then suggested to her that maybe her counts might be up this week too. Then, wow, the next day she hit 126! I love the power of suggestion! So now if her HGB is up again this next week then we can consider taking out her line!

There is so much more I want to type but I'm tired tonight. It's 11:30 already! So I'm going to copy the Facebook post I made so you can read it as well as the email update I received from Celeste's stepmom Michelle today. It's the first time she has ever suggested things for our Facebook group to focus their thoughts and prayers on. She is a member of the group but has never posted anything. I think it's a good sign. We've been getting along really well when we've been at appointments with Celeste the last few weeks.

Maybe I can call again next week. Celeste has an ultrasound on Monday and her next check-up is on Wednesday. My love, thoughts, and prayers are with you. Have a wonderful weekend! (Celeste comes home to me tomorrow morning so we will have a good weekend together as well.)

Always,
Laura

This week at Celeste's check-up appointment her blood counts are up again, but her weight is down. We had a long discussion about eating more and more frequently because the alternative is not fun. It would mean a feeding tube. Well, that did the job!

Once she got home she had made a huge effort to eat more. Please pray that every calorie will help her gain some of the lost pounds back and give her more strength as well. She's eating ice cream with her meals and having turkey soup even for breakfast sometimes and juices instead of just water. She really doesn't want that NG tube and I don't blame her.

Hayley is working on eating enough as well so she doesn't have to have it again. Please pray that both girls will develop good healthy appetites and will continue to get stronger and stronger.

The great news with the increase in Celeste's blood counts is that if her hemoglobin continues to go up next week then we can consider taking her central line out! That will also mean she won't have to have the enoxaparin shots that she hates getting in her arm. Please pray that her hemoglobin continues to rise to normal levels. Her HGB level was 109 when she went in to the hospital in July; we would love to see it rise to above 100 again.

Yesterday, Celeste had her first visit from one of her old school teachers who will be her tutor for the next few months. Her goal is to be well enough to go back to school in January! This evening she is having a special night out at a friend's birthday party. It's wonderful for her to start having some normalcy in her life again.

Thank you everyone for your thoughts and prayers. Our family is so very thankful. Celeste has been doing just great! She's started drinking more juice instead of just water, Fruitopia Fruit Integration. She'd tried a bunch of other juices before and didn't like them. She's been eating butterscotch ripple ice cream (had a scoop for lunch and a scoop for dinner yesterday) and turkey soup as well (bedtime snack and breakfast this morning), as well as apple slices and blue freezies. She reaaaaaalllyyy doesn't want to have an NG tube, although I've reassured her that, if it does happen, it's certainly not because she's not doing her best (we know she is) and that none of us will be disappointed in her at all (because she was worrying about disappointing us). I'll be taking her to a drive-thru flu shot clinic (for the immunologically compromised) next Saturday for her flu shot. The doctor encouraged all of us to get it. Oh, and she also said that, with regard to the starting enoxaparin, if her hemoglobin is still going up next week, we might be able to consider taking her line out instead—something for the group to focus thoughts and prayers on. Michelle

---

Oct 22, 2011

Oh Laura,

These girls are so amazing. I am so happy to see that they are really progressing almost exactly the same. We will talk about taking out Hayley's port after the big MRI on October 29 and her spinal tap on October 30. They are truly an inspiration, and I am so glad that Michelle and you seem to be more on the same page. God is good. I'm actually running out the door to help my brother move apartments, so we can email again during the week with more details. Praise God.

Laurie

———

Nov 2, 2011

Hi Laura,

Just checking in to see how you and Celeste are doing. Hayley and I were just talking about you and hoping things are going well for all of you. We were a little disappointed that Hayley's MRI didn't show much improvement, but we are staying the course and keeping the faith. Not much is new here. We have our lumbar puncture tomorrow. Hayley's appetite is better and she's getting more energy. We are still praying very hard for you and the situation about Celeste living in your home as well as complete healing of course.

Love and prayers forever,
Laurie

———

Nov 7, 2011

Hi Laurie

I think of you guys all the time. From your CarePages updates it really sounds like Hayley and Celeste are both doing the same things at the same time. Celeste gained a half-pound this last week. We were worried because she didn't eat as well that week, so we were telling her to think heavy thoughts and had her wear the heaviest track pants she owned so it wouldn't look like she had lost any weight! But she did OK and went up .3 of a kilogram.

I had Celeste and Desy and Connlan home for the weekend and cooked up a tonne of food, all their favorites to keep Celeste eating. We are hoping Celeste gets her central line taken out in about three weeks, at the end of November. The doctor wanted to keep it in for one more month in case they need it to give her antibiotics if she were to get a fever. But he doesn't know Celeste; she won't get a fever. But we still have to wait and then tell him "I told you so" at the end of the month. She had her flu shot last week. They have told us our whole family has to get the flu shot. I have never had one before. I don't get the flu, but, again, it's procedure.

Because she still has her line in and her platelet count has gone back up again she does have to have an anti-clotting needle every day again until the line comes. She had an ultrasound and an appointment with the thrombosis clinic about it all. Again I know she's going to be fine. She only got the clots because of the line, so it will be good to get that out soon.

I'm glad Hayley is getting her port out soon. Celeste can't wait to be able to lie on her stomach without lines and caps and stuff bothering her. When it does come out we are also hoping she can stay home with me for a week at a time between clinic appointments. It would be really nice.

Grayson misses her and she misses Grayson a lot. They were so cute cuddling together in bed Saturday night. He still doesn't understand why they only come home for two days and are gone for so long. Thank you for praying for our family. I know blessings are coming and things will work out soon. We got the results back on Celeste's MRI, her main tumour has shrunk 91 percent now, up from 84 percent in June. It hadn't changed at all in August so I know the feelings you have. Celeste's tumour is finally 1.4 centimetres x 1.5 centimetres x 1.4 centimetres, so it's finally down to the same size Hayley's started at right?

I know our girls are going to be just fine. Think of how far they have come already. Just remember to see Hayley as healthy and happy. Know that she is perfectly whole and then look for the evidence that supports that. See it, believe it, feel it in your heart, and wait patiently for the doctors to figure out what you have known all along.

I keep telling people that the last 9 percent of Celeste's tumour left could be just scar tissue; we don't know. If it stays the same, it's OK and it may continue shrinking over the next few months. As long as it isn't growing we're good. She is healing and getting stronger every day and it is the same with Hayley. Expect the good news because God has promised us the blessings, for our Heavenly

Father is a God of truth and goodness and mercy, and he loves us. See the good test results in your mind and know that soon the doctors will see those same test results in their hands.

Our daughters are being healed right now. Just like the leper whom the Savior commanded to go down to the river to bathe in order to be healed, so too must our daughters make their journey and trust that soon they too will be made clean and whole. "Now faith is the substance of things hoped for, the evidence of things not seen." Hebrews 11:1 (KJV)

My other good news is that an art gallery in Thorold, Ontario, is going to exhibit my paintings. My goal is to find two or three galleries that can exhibit them before next summer when I'll auction them to raise funds for Hayley, Sick Kids Hospital, and Ronald McDonald House. I am going to sell prints as well, as soon as they come back from the photographer, hopefully next week.

Celeste had a great time making stuff with Bendaroos with her sister and a friend who came over on the weekend. I got Matt to take pictures, so I'll upload them and send them to you in the next couple of days. I should go to bed now. I'm looking forward to hearing more good news soon. Oh, and I hope you guys don't lose your power too much more. I'm sure that gets to be a pain. It was because of snow wasn't it?

All my love,
Laura

―――――――

Nov 8, 2011

Oh Laura,

I am so happy to hear the good news about Celeste. That is just so fabulous. What an amazing girls she is. People from church as well as my friends and family always laugh, saying they think of Celeste as my other daughter because I always talk to them about Hayley and Celeste. They say that they can't imagine not hearing Celeste updates. Everyone here continually prays for your entire family.

We know in our hearts that Hayley and Celeste will be fine and will be a testament to God. He loves them, and they know it. So many people are coming to know Him through our girls. Sometimes I want to say, God, please leave these two beautiful girls alone and just let them heal, but I know he is healing them and it's all part of his plan. I am so amazed at the strength of the two of them. We really are lucky, Laura, to be their moms. I am so happy to hear that you got to have your whole family together. I truly believe it will happen more and more until you have everyone together all the time.

I'm so happy to hear about your paintings. You are probably the most talented person I know. I was so amazed at your paintings and your writing. To top it off you are a great cook and caregiver and a fabulous mom. You are such an inspiration to all of us, but especially me. I feel so blessed to have you in my life. Whenever I start to feel down, I think of you and remember that there will come a day when our two families will meet and realize that God put us together. Thank you for always being there for me with such encouragement. You are a blessing—a real blessing.

All my love,
Laurie

————————

Nov 15, 2011

Hi Laurie,

I'm so happy for Hayley today, getting her port out. I'm sure it will go smoothly and she will be back to normal in no time. Celeste can't wait to get her central line out. We had a miracle last week. The doctor had told us that she would have to wait until the end of November to get the line out, and then on Wednesday we were handed the date and time for her appointment for a consult with the surgeon. First they booked it with the original surgeon who put her first line in, (we weren't happy with his skills, she couldn't move her neck for weeks after the surgery) and the consult was for Dec 20 with no actual surgery scheduled. She'd probably have to wait until January to have it out.

Celeste was really disappointed and when the doctor and Michelle left the room, I asked her about how she was feeling and what would she like to happen. At first she said, "I don't know." I asked her if she would like it out by the end of the month because we could pray for a miracle.

She said yes, she'd like that. So I told her we'll pray for a miracle! Three hours later Michelle called me to say they had gotten an appointment with another surgeon for November 28 and the surgery is scheduled for Nov 29! I was so excited! Then I had to tell Michelle about the conversation I had with Celeste. I think Michelle is starting to believe in miracles now!

I love miracles and I love it when our Heavenly Father makes them happen so quickly! Celeste is really learning that miracles really do happen! These are lessons she will take with her for the rest of her life. Both she and Hayley will be able to accomplish big things because they will know so well how God answers prayers. There is no room there for doubt and they can teach others how to really believe and have faith!

Laurie, thank you for always saying such kind words. I admire you and your faith and ability to continually quote scriptures and tell everyone about God's grace and express your gratitude. You have raised such beautiful, well-adjusted, talented children. You are such a good mom. I'm so glad to have your example and to have you as my friend. I am so thankful our families were brought together to support each other in this way. To me, Celeste and Hayley really have become inseparable in my mind. I can't talk about Celeste without talking about Hayley too!

I shared your recent update so that everyone on our list could pray for Hayley today. This last week has been a wonderful week for me. My paintings are going to be exhibited for the whole month of December with the exhibit opening on Friday December 2! I wish you and your family could be there. I have named the exhibit *Two Girls, One Prayer*, same as the working title of the book. Everyone so far says it's just perfect. I'm going to tell the story of our girls to put up with the paintings.

Does Hayley have a favorite photo of herself I can use? I'm using her favorite painting, the one Hayley named *Waves*, on the publicity postcards and posters for the exhibit. All the paintings are now available on a website where anyone can view and purchase prints as well. http://tinyurl.com/qf5xy9u. My goal is to find a new gallery every month to exhibit in and raise more publicity for the auction next summer.

Lots of things to keep me busy between Celeste's appointments! Celeste will have her full MRI—brain and spine—in the next ten days. We're just waiting for a date. Please give Hayley a big hug for me. Let her know we bug Celeste about eating all the time too. She was down 3 pounds last week but we hope it was just a fluke. She's eating lots of chicken soup and lasagne tasted all right the other day. So maybe she can start eating her favorite food, spaghetti with sauce, soon. I'm so pleased to hear about Hayley's exciting news and activities. She's a very lucky girl. The most public place Celeste has been so far is the hospital and once to the video store! She's still on restrictions, including the low bacteria diet for another month, and then she can finally have restaurant food again!

'Peggy' from the Discovery Card commercials gave Celeste a shout-out in a picture on Facebook the other day. I had never seen the commercials before then but I watched a bunch on YouTube—hilarious! I have to run now. Matt's about to pick me up so we can go get Grayson from school, get the boys haircuts, and then tonight go out for dinner for Matt's birthday!

All my love,
Laura

————

Nov 16, 2011

Oh Laura,

That is just wonderful news. I'm so glad for Celeste that she's getting her central line out and for Michelle because she's realizing that God is working miracles in your lives. I'm so happy that you have such a strong faith. It's a huge part of my life, knowing that you believe that God is in control and is working in all of our lives. I can't imagine someone going through this without faith. You are a great mother. I know that at times you feel upset because the kids are not with you all of the time, but I feel it in my heart that they love you deeply and know that you love them and are truly WITH them all the time. When I hear about all of the cooking that you do and how excited you get when you see them, I know that they see your positive energy and love shining through.

You never have to doubt that you are a great mother.

Your positive love, energy, and faith are what have gotten Celeste through this horrendous ordeal. Never, ever doubt that you are a wonderful mother to Celeste and you are an inspiration to so many people. You continually amaze me with your talents and kindness. I am so excited for you about your paintings. You are unbelievably talented. I can't even draw a stick figure. I love the idea of two girls and one prayer. It's so true and appropriate.

Yes, Hayley is so excited about the Taylor Swift concert. She is really looking forward to it. She got her port out yesterday and is very sore today. Her throat is scratchy and she is having trouble lifting her arm because it pulls where the incision was made. They made the cut in the same scar so it's tender. They sewed it up with dissolvable stitches, surgical glue, and steri-strips. She's taking Tylenol today for the pain and is starting to feel a little better tonight. I hope she sleeps well. We will be thinking about you during the exhibit. Good luck.

Love,
Laurie

Nov 22, 2011

Hi Laurie,

We're at the hospital this week. Celeste's doctor has ordered an NG feeding tube. Last night was a hard adjustment for her. Maybe Hayley can Skype with her today. How is Hayley doing? Hopefully we can connect today.

Love,
Laura

Nov 26, 2011

Hi Laura,

Oh, I'm so sorry about the NG tube. As much as Celeste will hate it and it will take you time to figure out what and how much and what time to give it to her, it really works. I am thankful that we had it during Hayley's treatment. I sincerely think it helped her to be able to fight harder. Hayley has never been a good eater, but during this time, she barely ate anything. Hayley totally sympathizes with Celeste. We have been crazy busy here lately with Thanksgiving, etc., so I haven't checked messages. Hayley will send Celeste a Skype message today and Celeste can ask her questions. Hang in there. It is actually a wonderful thing and it's only temporary. I've been telling Hayley that she has to push herself more so we don't get another NG. She's trying, but it's so hard for them.

Love and prayers,
Laurie

Nov 28, 2011

Hi Laura,

I just wanted to check in with you to see how Celeste is doing with the NG tube. We had so much trouble regulating it for Hayley to find out how much and when to give it. We found that it was best to give her two cans when she woke up in the morning, one around 2:00 p.m. (or so), and then two cans just before bed or while she was sleeping. It helped her wake up feeling like she digested the cans.

Originally they wanted her to have all five cans together, but she threw up almost every day. We used Nutren 1.5. We tried the 2.0, but it was just too heavy for Hayley's stomach. Each can of the 1.5 has 375 calories. I know the girls were chatting a bit about the tube and Hayley feels for Celeste. Hayley truly hated it, but she knows that it really does help. She didn't mind its being in so much; it's just the placement and the embarrassment of walking around with it. A lot of kids place it down every night so they don't have to walk around during the day with it, but it was too stressful for Hayley to consider taking it out and putting it in every day.

You must be so excited about the exhibit!! We will be thinking about you constantly.

We hope you have a wonderful Christmas and New Year.

Love you guys,
Laurie

Dec 7, 2011

Dear Laura,

You and Celeste have been on our minds constantly. We are hoping that she is gaining weight and feeling better. Things here are good. Hayley is slowly getting back to normal (or as normal as possible). If you need anything, please let us know. Also, we hope that your opening went well. You are truly talented.

Laurie

———

Dec 12, 2011

Hi Laurie,

I have been thinking about you and Hayley every day. It has been such a busy two weeks. Celeste spent four days in the hospital getting her adjusted to her NG tube. The doctor set up the schedule of 80 milliliters an hour for twelve hours every night, receiving 960 milliliters total of "Jevity" throughout the night. It just took a few nights to increase her flow rate from 20 milliliters to 80 milliliters an hour. She then eats anything she wants all day.

I think it's working well because even being fed all night she is still hungry in the morning for breakfast.

Last week I spent two days in London for Celeste's appointment with the surgeon then her surgery to remove her line. It went really well and she didn't even need a stitch. Then I came back home to work and prepare for the art opening. It was a great night. I had lots of terrific feedback with lots inquiries into how both our girls are doing. Everyone is so pleased to hear they are doing so well. I had an interview on Monday and a few more interviews coming up. I will send you the link when the article is published.

I am so happy to hear Hayley has the go ahead to return to school in January. Celeste is hoping for the same. She has clinic today so hopefully we can find out today. I am hoping to see her MRI results today while I am here. Please give Hayley my love.

Love and prayers,
Laura

———————

Jan 10, 2012

Hi Laura,

I have been thinking of you and Celeste constantly. How did she handle going back to school? Hayley is doing great. We are so thankful that our Heavenly Father is taking care of our babies. Please know that you and Celeste are in our thoughts and prayers all the time. People here continually remind me that they are still praying for Celeste. I hope you are getting to see her more often.

Love,

Laurie

Jan 10, 2012

Hi Laurie,

I have been thinking of you and Hayley constantly as well. I tried to call a few times, I left a message on Saturday because I couldn't wait to hear how things went at school for Hayley. Celeste goes back for her first day today.

I had the kids home with me from December 30 to January 7. On the Friday, January 30, Celeste went to a church youth overnight activity. I was able to go as a chaperone. I read your post about the youth activity Hayley is attending this weekend. It sounds very similar. Celeste loved it. She participated in all the indoor workshops and once did the quarter-mile walk between main lodge and the residence building we stayed in. She and I were able to share a room so we could hook her up for her feed at night and she could rest by herself if she needed it. It was so pretty up north with all the snow.

Last Wednesday was her clinic day and she gained 5 pounds so we are starting to wean her off the feed, down to ten hours from twelve hours. I wish it was a faster wean, but maybe next week we can cut it in half to five hours or something, although she may need extra calories now that she's back to school and doing more.

THE ROAD TO RECOVERY

The whole month of December was really hard for me. It was like the whole year suddenly caught up with me. I felt shell-shocked. Have you experienced any of that? I held it together for so long, and then when I could finally relax a little it all came flooding at me. Christmas ended up just being very quiet with Matt and Grayson and me, and it was exactly what we needed. I don't think I left the house for three days! Then when the kids came home for New Year's we did lots of family stuff and had fun.

I read about your trip to Florida. That sounded wonderful. I'm so glad you were able to go and Hayley enjoyed it so much.

I have started talking to Celeste about which high school she will attend. We have a great school here that some of her old friends will be attending. I am hoping she will make a firm decision that she wants to live here in September. Once she has made her decision I can start working on the paperwork so she can move back. Our schools here will be having their open houses soon. Will Hayley be choosing her high school soon too? I am so thankful that life is going back to normal for them. We are so blessed.

This year has been such a whirlwind. I couldn't have gotten through it all without the Lord and the blessing of finding you and your family. Do you have plans for March and spring break yet? Maybe we could drive down to New Jersey to see you, so the girls can finally meet. It would depend on when the school boards schedule the breaks, but maybe we could come for a weekend if the weeks don't match.

Hayley mentioned on Skype being in the school play. When will be the performances? We're signing Celeste back into our local theater group's youth acting classes again starting this month. She won't be able to do this year's play because of schedules at her dad's but hopefully next year she'll be back with me so she can perform in the next play. This year's classes include acting for film and TV, so we may be finding her a local agent if she really enjoys it.

Make A Wish Foundation was not able to grant Celeste's wish to meet the actors in England for the *Doctor Who* TV show, so it looks I will working on that one myself. I told her I will make sure she gets that wish even if they couldn't arrange it. So I will use all our theater connections to make sure it happens! What is Hayley's wish?

Celeste has her next MRI scheduled for Jan 23. I can't wait to see how much more is gone. She only has 9 percent of her original tumour left. When does Hayley have her next MRI? Her three months should be soon right?

I painted twenty-four more paintings in December and finished the one I had started with Hayley's colours back in the summer. I had one painting that just wasn't quite right but now it is done. I'll attach a copy for you to see. I hope Hayley likes it.

If you are ever on Facebook or your husband is, you can see all the sneak peeks on my (fan) page. It's a public page, and I don't think you have to log in to see it. https://www.facebook.com/LauraLaneAuthorPoetArtist There are links to the newspaper articles from last month as well.

Everyone keeps asking about Hayley. I am so glad I can share the story of our amazing girls and their awesome faith. I want to start putting together all our emails and online posts so I can have the book written and published by this summer. If you know of anyone in the publishing industry who would be interested in the story of our girls, please let me know so I can send off submissions to them.

I have so much to tell you to catch up on all the emails that I thought about but didn't have the energy to write in December. OK, I'm sending this off now.

With love and gratitude,
Laura

———————

Jan 10, 2012

Hi Laura,

That's so wonderful that Celeste has gained weight. I know she will be off the tube soon. I totally understand what you are saying. I've been on such a crazy whirlwind. I just feel so exhausted all of the time. I think it's just catching up with both of us. We're not as young as we used to be and these ordeals have just been unreal. I was thinking about our retreat this weekend. That was the last thing Hayley did last year before she was admitted to the hospital in January. These girls are so amazing. Yes, we drove down to Florida. It was actually exhausting. I didn't really want to go because it's a twenty-four-hour drive each way and we could only stay there for four and a half days.

Anthony really wanted to go, so I gave in. Hayley was worried about feeling nauseous, but she did well and it was good to get so much fresh air. We are supposed to go to Minnesota to Taylor's school during Easter break, but I'm not sure. When is your break? It would be so good to see you and for the girls to actually meet. Your paintings are just amazing. You really are talented. Yes, Hayley and Taylor have always been in plays and always have been singing. That's great that Celeste does them too. I don't have any details about the play yet. Hopefully she will get some info from school. It's so good to hear from you. Please let me know how Celeste did with school.

Laurie

———————

Jan 19, 2012

Hi Laura,

We have been thinking of you and Celeste so much lately. We are hoping that she is doing well now that she is back to school. Is she getting tired? Hayley is doing well, but she is struggling in math somewhat. Most of her other subjects are fine, but she lost so much of math that she is getting frustrated when she doesn't understand something. I've been sitting with her to start from the beginning and basics of algebra to make sure she understands the fundamentals. We have four levels of math in eighth grade in our schools. Hayley is in the third level, which is Algebra I and II. She wants to switch to just Algebra I, but her teachers feel that she belongs in her class.

I've been in touch with the teachers, and I've told them that I agree with them, but now I need to get Hayley to agree so she doesn't get upset.

I'm trying hard not to get nervous about our MRI on January 28, but it's hard. One minute I completely trust that she will be fine and we will get great results, and then I panic in the next moment. I get so annoyed at myself because you really can't live like that. It does no one any good, but I guess it's just natural. I don't know about you, but I feel like I will never be able to completely rest because I know that she will have these tests forever.

Anthony and I have been asked to speak at CHOP in March for a parents' forum for newly diagnosed patients and their families. We are supposed to talk of Hayley's diagnosis, how we felt, what confused us, what helped, and anything else that we think will help a new family. Then they want Hayley and the other kids to speak to the patients and siblings. Hayley wants to do it, but Taylor and Matthew really want nothing to do with it. They want to get their lives back and not allow cancer to have any more power. I respect their decision, and sometimes I agree too. I'm tired of cancer. It seems to be everywhere.

I hope you are doing well and not feeling so exhausted anymore. I still feel really tired all the time. I'm taking some new vitamins and hoping that will help a bit. Say hi to Celeste for us!

Love and prayers always,
Laurie

———————

Jan 24, 2012

Laura,

I'm up at church right now working on stuff for our high school retreat, and I just wanted to check in with you. I know Celeste had her MRI yesterday, and I'm dying to know how you and she are doing. We have been praying like crazy for her. Our group at church just finished praying for Celeste, so I grabbed a computer and decided to check in with you. Praying, praying, praying.

Laurie

———————

Jan 31, 2012

Hi Laurie,

I am so happy to hear about Hayley! That's wonderful! I am so thankful that all of our prayers continue to be answered! Celeste has been off her feeding tube for a week now. She threw up last Tuesday and really didn't want it to go back in again so they worked it out that if she drank a litre of chocolate milk every day it would be the same number of calories. So as long as she weighs herself every couple of days to make sure she isn't losing (her weight is remaining stable) then she should be fine without the tube!

I had a great weekend with her and Connlan this weekend and Celeste told me she definitely wants to move back in time to start high school here in September! I let her know that as far as the courts are concerned that she is old enough to choose, especially now that she will be starting high school. She really misses her little brother, Grayson. He really misses her and Connlan and Desiree too. They cuddle a lot and he likes to sleep in the girls' room when they come home for the weekend.

I really enjoyed all the cuddles all weekend too. I am so thankful for all those nights in hospital when I got to climb into Celeste's bed and hold her until she fell asleep. I wouldn't give up those nights for anything. It was our little bit of heaven, of peace, during the storm.

I know I have struggled to develop patience during this long year, but this last week I read a quote by Henri Nouwen:

"Patience is a hard discipline. It is not just waiting until something happens over which we have no control: the arrival of the bus, the end of the rain, the return of a friend, the resolution of a conflict. Patience is not waiting passively until someone else does something. Patience asks us to live the moment to the fullest, to be completely present in the moment, to taste the here and now, to be where we are. When we are impatient we try to get away from where we are. We behave as if the real thing will happen tomorrow, later, and somewhere else. Let's be patient and trust that the treasure we look for is hidden in the ground on which we stand."

I think this year I have learned to appreciate every moment more than I ever have in the past. I know today I am so thankful for today's moment of rejoicing in today's blessing. Please hug Hayley for me and ask her to hug you for me as well.

All my love and prayers,
Laura

———————

Feb 1, 2012

Oh Laura,

I am sitting here with tears of joy in my eyes. I am so happy that Celeste has come to this decision. You need her, and she needs you. I really believe that your time of cuddling in bed in the hospital (we did it all the time) has really been what she needed to make that decision. When do you think she will come home to you? The summer? Grayson is going to be so happy to have one of his big sisters home with him. Do you think the other two will consider coming home or are they just too involved in their lives since they are older? I think that it's harder the older they get to change their lives. Oh, I am so happy for you. We pray about it all the time. I can't wait to tell Hayley that Celeste is coming home. She said she could really tell that Celeste misses you when she leaves the hospital and goes to her dad's house. She said that Celeste always looked down when she talked about it. I love that quote you sent. I really think our situations have helped us to realize how lucky we are every minute of our lives and to always give thanks.

Hayley is doing really well. We are both so lucky that this treatment seems to have worked for our babies. Our doctor told us that they are closing out the St. Jude's protocol now to gather the data for how well it worked. I guess we are lucky that they got diagnosed last year.

Laura, we will keep praying for strength for Celeste to tell her dad. Praying, praying, praying.

Love and tons of hugs and prayers,
Laurie

———

Feb 21, 2012

Hi Laura,

I was just thinking about you and Celeste, so I thought before things got crazy here, I would check in to see how things are going. Things here are going well. Hayley is feeling better and better. She's completely off of her meds now. She's no longer taking anti-nausea pills (Zofran) and she's feeling good. She's eating so well now, but the weight comes on very, very slowly. She's still not at school full time, but we're getting closer. We added another class last week, so I'm basically taking her home for a good lunch and she's only missing one class plus the lunch class. Her hair is slowly coming back. She's frustrated because there are spots that don't seem to be coming back. Her hair is coming in darker and it looks a little curly. Her hair used to be blonde and very straight. How is Celeste doing in that department? We've been praying hard about your ex accepting that Celeste wants to go to school by you. How is that going? Also, how is your art show going? Taylor came in for the weekend (thank you, Grandma and Grandpa) to go to a church retreat. Hope all is going well with you.

Love and prayers,
Laurie

———————

Feb 22, 2012

Hi Laurie,

I am so glad to hear about Hayley! Celeste has been going to school full time but her classes start later and she sits out gym classes and stays indoors for recess and lunches. There are a couple of girls who have permission to stay in with her and they play board games instead of going outside. Her school is kindergarten to grade eight. She is still wearing her walking splints to help strengthen her tendons but is walking well.

Celeste's hair is exactly the same. Some bare patches still, very dark—it almost looks black—and curly. Her hair was light brown before and straight. But I think it might be kind of like when they were babies: sort of downy hair that first grows in, and then it changes as they get older. I have a feeling it will be like that this time for them.

My good friend is a master stylist and she was suggesting to Celeste if she shaved it right back down again it would grow in thicker. Celeste wasn't ready to do that yet. She was too pleased about the growth she has—a symbol of how far she has come along since last summer! I'm sure Hayley can understand. But as it grows and they do have haircuts or trims it will grow in thicker and stronger and I'm sure with the sunlight this spring and summer it will lighten up again too.

Celeste told me again she doesn't know now about moving back. Her dad is telling her again she can't because her doctor is in London. I know by next fall she will only be going for check-ups once every two or three months, or longer. It's heartbreaking to me that he tells her things like that, but when I had a blessing to comfort me I was told to trust the Lord and be patient.

Proverbs 3:5–6: "Trust in the Lord with all thine heart; and lean not unto thine own understanding. In all thy ways acknowledge him, and he shall direct thy paths." (KJV)

So I am focusing on my artwork and the auction next summer. My paintings were in the Fonthill Library for the month of January and on Feb 10 we had a grand opening for a new gallery that will feature my paintings for the month of February.

I started the week doing my first ever talk show interview about my book, poetry, art, and work as a LifeSuccess consultant. I collected more than $700 in orders for my greeting cards on the Monday, spent Tuesday running around ordering and packaging up 100 sets of cards, and then drove to Toronto to deliver the cards and in the end sold more than 100 sets. At 3:00 p.m. I got a phone call that I had won a contest I entered, a trip for two to Sandals all-inclusive resort in Antigua in the Caribbean! I entered two weeks ago by posting a video answering the question: Why do my Valentine and I deserve a trip to Sandals Grande Antigua, so I told them about our last year and that's why Matt and I deserve a trip. We won!

I'm going to paint some more paintings, and I'm asking other artists to donate pieces. My goal is to find fifty artists who will donate to the auction. Yesterday I had a TV news interview and another interview and photo shoot for the paper in St. Catharine's.

Our trials temper us spiritually just as fire tempers steel. It is our willingness to submit to our trials and know that the Lord sees within us something beautiful and he will continue to strengthen us as we are tempered in the fire of our trials. The ladies at church all keep saying, "Laura, you just don't know how to have a boring life, do you?" If it doesn't kill you, it makes you stronger!

I have offered to the many different grade eight classes who know Celeste that if they want to sell the greeting card sets as a fundraiser for their grade eight end-of-year class trips or graduation parties that they receive 25 percent from the sale of the cards. If Hayley's class needs to raise funds as well I would be pleased to speak to her teachers about it. And if whoever is still organizing fundraising for your family would like cards to sell as well just let me know and I'll send down as many sets as they would like. It's a set of six cards (six different images) including Hayley's favorite *Waves* and Celeste's, *Flowers for Celeste.*

As you have probably guessed or noticed I am determined to find the silver lining in the last year and turn all our lemons into lemonade. At the rate things are going, once the book I am writing about the girls is finished, we will have such a huge inspiring story it will make it on Oprah's book club list and we can share the miracle of prayers, faith, and trusting in the Lord to the world! I hope we can finally get together soon. My kids are with me for March break March 9–16. Do any of those days work around the days you are going out to see Taylor? How is Taylor enjoying college? Does Hayley miss her a lot?

I hope you have a wonderful week. I pray that your life has less drama than mine has had lately although I wish you could win a nice trip like we did! Thank you so much for your prayers as well.

With all my love and prayers as well,
Laura

———

Feb 22, 2012

Oh Laura,

You are the most positive person I've ever met, and I agree 100 percent that good always comes out of bad. It's so sad about your ex trying to convince Celeste to stay where she is. He should really think about what's best for her. I love that verse and always try to live by that as well. My problem is that I lack patience usually, but I'm learning little by little. I would love to get together with you, but our break is in April instead of March. Maybe we could try during the summer break instead. We will keep you all in our prayers as usual. Give Celeste a big hug for us when you see her.

Love and prayers,
Laurie

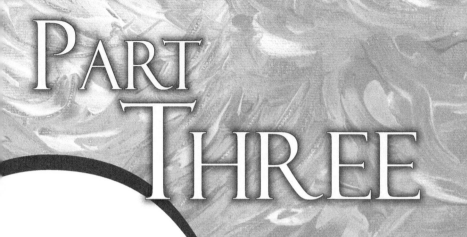

PART
THREE

> *"Hope is important because it can make the present moment less difficult to bear. If we believe that tomorrow will be better, we can bear a hardship today."*
>
> THICH NHAT HANH

Chapter 8

REACH OUT AND CONNECT

Just four months before Celeste was diagnosed, I was in West Palm Beach, Florida, taking Bob Proctor's five-day training course to become a Certified LifeSuccess Consultant. For the training we had to become proficient in teaching others how our mind works, understanding the conscious and subconscious mind.

I had been preparing my presentation for months. I listened to Bob's materials over and over again until I really understood how my thoughts controlled my feelings, which controlled my actions. This all led to the results in my life. A great deal stems from whether we focus on negative or positive thoughts and emotions. Negative thoughts and emotions produce negative results and positive thoughts and emotions produce positive results.

I also learned that negative thoughts like worry, doubt, and fear, stem from some form of ignorance or lack of knowledge. If I was afraid it usually meant I lacked knowledge. If I was worrying about something, in order to turn it around I just needed to find out what knowledge I was missing. Once you have the bigger picture—the missing information, understanding, or knowledge—you then can stand in a position of hope and confidence and can function with renewed strength and courage.

I had no idea then how much I was about to put this newfound knowledge into practice.

Once Celeste was diagnosed, each time a wave of doubt or fear would come over me, I would ask myself, "What is it that I don't know?" When I was scared by what was happening to Celeste, I would ask questions or read up on her diagnosis to better understand and that took away the fear.

I knew I was going to have to be at my strongest in order to best help her. That's when I realized I wouldn't be able to do this on my own. I was going to need help.

Looking back now three years later, I can see the steps we (our family and Hayley and Laurie's family) took to get through the new and frightening diagnosis, the long and multiple treatments, the recovery process, the relapses and the need to refocus our thoughts when things turned bad. There were five keys things that Laurie and I did that helped to foster hope, and these things ultimately gave us the strength and courage to continue on every day. We share these with you so you too can feel that hope, feel that strength and feel that courage.

We realized we had to reach out, connect, reflect, express, and love.

Reach out

No matter how strong or independent you are, you can't do this alone. You have to reach out.

Once I received the initial news that Celeste was going in for an MRI and would soon be going in for surgery, I made those first few calls to family and church members immediately. I knew there were several things we needed right then. A place in London for Matt and Grayson to stay overnight while I was with Celeste. A priesthood blessing for Celeste from the bishop. Later that night I sent out an initial post on Facebook letting people know what was going on and asking them to pray for Celeste.

When we began to process the magnitude of her diagnosis, I knew I was going to need even more help. I created a dream list, the best of the best in their different areas of expertise, and told them that I would be so grateful if I could receive their help. These were people who could help me be at my best so I could strong enough to help Celeste.

I called or emailed each one to ask their advice or ask for referrals to who was the best person to see in the Toronto area. I spoke to church leaders, to EFT practitioners, transformational leaders, and healers. I bought the books that were suggested to me and found more on my own. I was willing to ask anyone and everyone I could think of who could help me and, ultimately, Celeste.

Once Celeste started her treatments, I created a Facebook group to keep people updated. Laurie created a CarePages page for Hayley. Laurie reached out to her church community and their large extended family in New Jersey. This became a huge support to each of us, knowing we weren't alone. This is how we found each other.

I had found a website dedicated to educating people about pineoblastoma, created by a mom, Stacy, who had lost her little boy Wade in 2010 (www.pineoblastoma.com). On that website she has a page dedicated to listing other children diagnosed with pineoblastoma.

As I scrolled through, I saw the listing for another little girl, Hayley, who was the same age as Celeste and was diagnosed the same month. I couldn't believe it. Someone else was going through the same thing at the same time as us. I found her on CarePages and reached out to her and her family. It was such a blessing to find each other.

Reaching out can also be the source of peace, comfort, and happiness for ourselves and our children. The dream list I made included Bob Proctor, Jack Canfield, Hale Dwoskin, Carol Look, Michael Beckwith, President Thomas S. Monson, Nick Vujicic and Adam McLeod—Dream Healer. Bob Proctor spoke with me and gave me guidance. Jack Canfield emailed me books he recommended I read and referred me to excellent healers. Hale Dwoskin referred me to his top Sedona Method practitioners in Toronto. Carol Look spoke with me and referred me to the perfect EFT practitioner in my area, Vivian Cannataro, who became my lifeline over the next couple of years.

Friends connected me with people from Michael Beckwith's church, Agape, and they included Celeste's name in the prayer list and sent a very beautiful prayer for her. We were able to arrange for Celeste to meet President Monson and he let her know that he was praying for her every day. A year and a half later, his office called to let her know that he still prayed for her daily. Kara from Nick Vujicic's office let me know that they would pray for Celeste, and Adam McLeod shared with me some great visualization techniques to use with Celeste. It is incredible how many people are willing to help if you just ask.

Once Celeste started her chemo, she needed some cheering up, so I contacted the CBC and Stuart McLean and his radio show the *Vinyl Café*—one of Celeste's favorite shows! Stuart and his staff wrote back and sent Celeste some of his CDs and books. I contacted one of her favorite Canadian bands, Chic Gamine. Band members Andrina Turenne and Alex Dirks arranged to call Celeste and sent her a signed copy of their newest CD and a poster for her room.

Celeste desperately wanted to see the new Pooh Bear movie when it came out in July 2011. We arranged to have the whole theater to ourselves (just our family) so she could watch it on the big screen. The incredible staff at the cinema welcomed Celeste and gave her loads of promotional gifts. It made it a terrific day for her, for our whole family.

To help me through the difficult months while Celeste was in the hospital, I reached out to the Therapeutic Touch Network of Ontario. They arranged for a lovely team of recognized practitioners to come to the hospital and provide me with Therapeutic Touch sessions every week over the months we were there. They also connected us with the hospital chaplain, who was a practitioner as well and could come to Celeste's room more often to help ease Celeste's discomfort between chemo treatments.

The biggest support Laurie received during Hayley's long months in the hospital was the love and support of her extended family. Their wonderful family members and friends stepped up to the challenge to practically run the house back home, looking after Anthony, Taylor, and Matthew so Laurie could put her full focus on Hayley. Meals and cleaning were taken care of, rides and visiting schedules were arranged, and then donations and fundraising were organized. It was a huge "Team Hayley" effort. But it first started out by reaching out to family and being willing to allow others to help.

Yes, it can be hard sometimes to allow others to serve you. Please let them. It is a gift and you both end up receiving.

While Hayley was in hospital, Laurie made the call to Annika Sorenstam, one of the top female golf professionals in the world, and asked if she would mind calling Hayley to cheer her up. Hayley loves golf and was thrilled to chat with Annika via Skype. They got along so famously that Annika offered to call Hayley every month to chat. Three years later, they still chat and have developed a wonderfully close relationship.

These are just some of the wonderful things that can happen when you reach out. You will have to choose who you reach out to. Not everyone you reach out to will be the perfect connection but it becomes the first step in making a connection. That's when miracles really start to happen.

Connect

The second step occurred naturally in consequence to reaching out. Once I found Laurie we began creating a beautiful connection between us. We had similar beliefs and attitudes and our girls were the same age so we had similar concerns about their development. We also had other children close in age.

As you read in the previous chapters, it didn't happen overnight but very quickly we were loving and supporting each other. Today we are nearly family, we feel so close. We celebrated and cried together, supported one another when we took turns being down and worried. It is the most blessed gift that has come about during this long ordeal. It required trusting and being vulnerable. It required admitting we needed help and that we couldn't do it alone.

During the long hours of waiting during doctor's appointments and hospital stays, I read and watched TED talks. One of my favorite authors and speakers is Brené Brown. She taught me a great deal about vulnerability and connection. In her book *Daring Greatly* she explains, "Connection is why we are here; we are hardwired to connect with others; it's what gives purpose and meaning to our lives, and without it there is suffering."

What I learned from her is that in order to have connection we must be willing to be vulnerable. The gift that comes from the courage of being vulnerable is that it begets "love, belonging, joy, courage, empathy, and creativity." She very poignantly points out that vulnerability is "the source of hope."

It gave me a great sense of hope knowing we weren't alone. Laurie and I finally had someone who understood our fears and was praying just as fervently for miracles. Celeste and Hayley now had someone who understood exactly what it felt like to be poked and prodded and had the same scars and knew what it felt like to be cooped up in a hospital room away from family and friends for days and weeks.

In Brené Brown's words "Vulnerability begets vulnerability: Courage is contagious . . . [One] act of vulnerability is predictably perceived as courageous by [others] and inspires others to follow suit." The circle of influence you have as you reach out and connect may have a ripple effect around, encouraging family, friends, and other parents to courageously do the same and reap the gifts that occur: love, belonging, and connection. That is when you can recognize that there is much to be grateful for when we allow these gifts and blessings into our lives.

Still it's not easy. In her book, The Gifts of Imperfection, Brown explains:

"One of the greatest barriers to connection is the cultural importance we place on 'going it alone.' Somehow we've come to equate success with not needing anyone. Many of us are willing to extend a helping hand, but we're very reluctant to reach out for help when we need it ourselves. It's as if we've divided the world into 'those who offer help' and 'those who need help.' The truth is that we are both."

Please let me reiterate here: You can't do this alone. Your child isn't doing this alone and nor do you have to. There is no shame in asking for help; it is one the most courageous things you'll ever do and will lead to greater connection with those around you.

Many times I found it difficult to ask for help for myself but I was willing to do so for my daughter. When I put together my dream list, I was finally willing to do for her what I, for many years, put off doing for myself. What I found most amazing was how many people were willing to help and wanted to connect and support me and my family. It was incredible. Today I feel so much more love and gratitude and connection than I ever did before and have some very terrific people in my life that I didn't before. These were the blessing for me in learning to reach out and allowing meaningful connections to occur. It gave me much to reflect on in my life.

> *"Strength does not come from physical capacity.*
> *It comes from an indomitable will."*

MAHATMA GANDHI

Chapter 9

REFLECT

Reflect

It is in the quiet moments of reflection that we can gain a greater feeling of hope when we remember and recognize all the positive things that are happening during this time of great difficulty.

When I started compiling my list of people I needed and wanted to contact, it was amazing to see how many people there actually were who were loving and supporting us. The outpouring of love was incredible, especially the numbers of people who were praying for Celeste and Hayley all over the world.

In Celeste's room, we took yellow and purple and flowered sticky notes and wrote every note of encouragement and love that was sent to Celeste. We listed every person who was praying for her and where in the world they were: Australia, England, France, the Netherlands, Norway, Sweden, Estonia, Romania, Ukraine,

Dubai, Hong Kong, all over Canada, and the United States. She was literally surrounded with love and prayers.

In Hayley's room, she had a huge map of the world with pins on it for all the places people were praying for her. Prayer circles and congregations and temples had both girls on their prayer rolls. It was so comforting to know our girls were so well loved and we had so many people praying for the miracles we desired to see. We had so much to be grateful for.

As a student of Bob Proctor, I showed him that I already had a good, solid understanding of prayer and energy and that I was doing all the right things for my girl. He gave me advice and readings, and a quote by Reverend Michael Beckwith. It's actually one of my favorite quotes and I had been living by its advice for the last year:

When anything happens:

1. It is what it is. Accept it. You cannot change it. It will either control you or, you will control it.

2. Harvest the good. The more you look for it, the more you'll find.

3. Forgive all of the rest. Forgive means to let go of completely, abandon.

4. I love that advice "Accept it, harvest the good, and forgive all the rest." It allows me to feel so much more at peace with difficult situations.

What Laurie and I discovered as one of the most difficult challenges was the weight of the decisions that needed to be made. We fervently prayed to know what we should be doing at each moment, each day, and each step of the way to best help our daughters.

If ever we needed inspiration from God, it was during this time.

After Celeste started chemo, a friend suggested a book by Joe Vitale and Dr. Ihaleakala Hew Len, *Zero Limits: The Secret Hawaiian System for Wealth, Health, Peace and More*. She felt strongly that it was book I needed to read.

This book featured the ancient Hawaiian teaching of Ho'oponopono. It's a long name for a beautiful and simple concept. It was exactly what I needed to learn to help me be better in tune with God so I could be open to the inspiration I so desperately needed as I sat with my daughter each day.

After reading all about Ho'oponopono, and learning all that Joe Vitale and Dr. Len had to share about the topic, I began to see what was hindering me from being connected to God and spirit and my ability to gain the inspiration I desperately needed to best care for Celeste.

First, I was reminded that God is love.

In each moment, He loves us. When we can connect to that feeling of love in the present moment, then we can connect to God and be open to the inspiration, to the guidance He wishes to give us in that moment.

When we recognize and accept our true identity, our relationship to God as one of His children, we then recognize our divine nature. We acknowledge that He really is in charge. He controls all things and He desires what is best for us. He loves us.

Problems occur when we focus not on the present moment but instead get caught up in the past. We get stuck in old memories, old beliefs and paradigms, and all the negative emotions of the past: resentment, fear, anger, blame, confusion, jealousy, hatred, and judgement.

It is at that point that we deny our true identity. We disconnect from God and inspiration is blocked. Our paradigms, beliefs,

TWO MOTHERS ONE PRAYER

and old memories are in charge. When we accept our true identity, when we are connected to God and spirit, when we are open to receiving inspiration, we are then feeling God's love, feeling grateful, loving, peaceful, kind, humble, fully responsible for our lives, and accepting of others.

So the key question is: how do we get back to feeling love and peace? How can we be open to inspiration when we are stuck in the emotions of fear and resentment and anger? We can't just say, "Be at peace!" We need to make a transition, and that is where the process of Ho'oponopono comes in.

In its most basic form, Ho'oponopono means: I'm sorry. Please forgive me. Thank you. I love you.

You have a silent conversation with God and say, "I'm sorry I'm stuck right now feeling (fear, resentment, anger, blame, etc.) for this situation, this person, this problem. Please forgive me." Then allow yourself to feel the peace and say "thank you" and "I love you" until you begin to feel the love in your heart again.

This process became a life-saver for me. There were many days when I had to sit across the room from my ex-husband and I would stew in the emotions of resentment and anger and frustration and blame. It would eat me up inside.

But once I began using the Ho'oponopono, I could have those silent conversations with God and say "I'm sorry I feel resentment toward David or Michelle right now. Please forgive me. Thank you. I love you." Now, many times, the feeling would come back as soon as I looked at my ex again, but I would just repeat those phrases over and over again until I could finally look at him without feeling the resentment.

Because the truth was that in that present moment he wasn't actually doing anything to me. He was just sitting there, but I was caught up in the past, remembering things that had happened years ago. The Ho'oponopono helped me to come back to the present moment and be grounded and feel the love God has for me and be open to the inspiration I needed to best help Celeste in the present moment. It brought me an incredible sense of peace.

I believe that peace is one of the key reasons we need to take the time to reflect. We make far better decisions when we are in a peaceful state. When your child is sick, there are so many important decisions that need to be made and for which you will need as much inspiration you can get. It is also one of the craziest and most stressful times you will ever experience.

Reflecting led to finding the peace to be open to the inspiration we needed. We learned to let go of the stress and worries, and we could focus on being there to best support our girls.

Two other resources and practices that we learned were the importance of getting away, even if just for small breaks, and learning to take the time for quiet contemplation or meditation.

Three months after Celeste was diagnosed, when she had just completed her radiation treatments, I took two days to get away to a cabin just a couple of hours drive north of our home. I took all the books and binders the hospital had given me, and all the information I had to digest about Celeste's diagnosis and treatment. I alternated between reading and studying, and taking breaks to visit the local spa. My little getaway renewed and refreshed me.

Laurie and her family have done this many times over the last few years. It's good for you, the mom and caregiver, to get away and it's good if the patient can get away too.

Laurie and her sister and Hayley took a couple of days to drive to Florida to spend a few days with her grandma at her place near the beach. All the sunshine and warm air did them a world of good, increasing Hayley's blood counts and lowering Laurie's blood pressure. They all needed the break and time to reflect.

Another way to make time and have small breaks can be as simple as going for a walk around the hallways of the hospital. The Toronto Sick Kids Hospital has a beautiful open atrium that extends from the lobby up to the ninth floor, bathing the whole area in light and sounds from a waterfall near the elevators that can be heard throughout the whole area. Each family room and play area for the four wings on every floor look out on the atrium as well. It became a great place to sit quietly and relax when I just needed a short break.

Another resource was the hospital chapel. I contacted the local Therapeutic Touch (TT) practice group and members were kind enough to come to the hospital weekly to provide me with twenty-minute TT sessions.

Therapeutic Touch is a healing energy modality practiced by many nurses to relieve pain and reduce stress. Our hospital chaplain was a TT practitioner and she worked on Celeste every week and the other practitioners would work with me on alternate weeks. We would use the chapel space for our quiet sessions. Some days I would see others parents coming into the chapel for daily prayers or simply to meditate. For those twenty minutes while I sat there with my eyes closed, I would reflect and meditate as well.

There is so much good that comes physically, emotionally, mentally, and spiritually from meditating and taking the time to quietly reflect on things. It helps us to open up to the big picture of what we are going through, helps us to find a bigger divine perspective.

During this time, one of the books that I was drawn to was Dr. Gerome Groupman's book, *The Anatomy of Hope,* and the biggest lesson I learned was a clearer definition of hope. I am paraphrasing and explaining this as I understand it: Hope is when we have a beautiful vision of something and a positive emotion to go along with it. When our world comes crashing down, when we are trapped in a deep, dark, despairing hopelessness, we need a bigger perspective. Hope comes when we reflect on all that we hold dear and true, when we acknowledge a higher power, when we acknowledge God in our lives and begin to see what He has planned for our lives.

You need to be able to find hope in your circumstances. We need it for ourselves and our children. Laurie and I both believe that when we reflect on all that we have and all that we love and all that we are thankful for, we feel that hope and that peace. We feel God keeping us buoyed up. We are able to face the challenges.

Yes, you are busy. And because of that, you need to take quiet time for reflection. That quiet time will help keep you grounded through all the busy minutes and challenging decisions that come along in any given day.

Tied into the act of reflecting is also the importance of taking the time to express.

"Vulnerability sounds like truth and feels like courage."

BRENE BROWN

Chapter 10

EXPRESS

Celeste had started her first round of chemo and she had thrown up countless times. Each time she threw up, I held the little bucket for her, wiped her face, handed her a cup of water, put that bucket aside, and reached for a new one. We washed, rinsed, and repeated all day.

The smell in her room was less than pleasant. This particular day, I hadn't eaten much at all. I was now feeling weak and nauseated from the stress and the smell. I felt so bad. I felt terrible for Celeste, yet I didn't know how I was going to handle this for four to six months.

When the nurses came in to tend to Celeste, I slipped out of the room and walked down to the nurse's station. I pulled Linh, our favorite nurse, aside and told her how I was feeling. I needed to know it was normal.

Linh hugged me and assured me it was OK to feel that way. With tears in my eyes, I thanked her. She encouraged me to take a little break and have some dinner.

I just needed someone to talk to, reassure me, and help me build my strength back up to keep going. This is such an important step in coping. You cannot do it alone and you cannot keep it all bottled up inside. Reach out. Connect. Reflect. Express.

You have to have find ways to express all that is going on within you.

It is essential that you express and let go of all the emotions that come up during this difficult time. This can also be one of the hardest things to do.

Expressing requires allowing yourself to be vulnerable. It requires sharing what is in our hearts and minds, and that takes courage. Brené Brown, in *The Gifts of Imperfection*, talks a great deal about courage. She explains: "The root of the word *courage* is *cor*—the Latin word for heart. In one of its earliest forms, the word *courage* had a very different definition than it does today. Courage originally meant 'To speak one's mind by telling all one's heart.' . . . that speaking honestly and openly about who we are, about what we're feeling, and about our experiences (good and bad) is the definition of courage."

It has taken courage to write this book and share our experiences with everyone, but even harder for me was expressing in my journal all the emotions I was feeling at the time. Some days I could do it and some days (for many months), I couldn't.

I had to find other ways to express how I was feeling. Some days I prayed my heart out and others I cried my eyes out. Other days I found someone to talk to, and many times I couldn't wait to talk to Laurie on the phone because I knew she understood.

No matter which way I expressed my feelings, frustrations, and fears, it always felt better afterward. I also learned it's important to find the right person for the job.

Barry Goldman explains in an *LA Times* article how to best know whom to share your frustrations with when dealing with delicate situations. He calls it the "'Ring Theory' of kvetching."

Kvetching means to complain (I had to look it up!). He explains that the "first rule is comfort in, dump out." When his wife, Susan, developed breast cancer, she developed a theory on who was allowed to complain to whom. It works like this:

> "Draw a circle. This is the center ring. In it, put the name of the person at the center of the current trauma. Now draw a larger circle around the first one. In that ring put the name of the person next closest to the trauma . . . Repeat the process as many times as you need to.

> "In each larger ring, put the next closest people. Parents and children before more distant relatives. Intimate friends in smaller rings, less intimate friends in larger ones. When you are done, you have a Kvetching Order.

> "Here are the rules. The person in the center ring can say anything she wants to anyone, anywhere. She can kvetch and complain and whine and moan and curse the heavens and say, 'Life is unfair' and 'Why me?' That's the one payoff for being in the center ring.

> "Everyone else can say those things too, but only to people in larger rings.

> "When you are talking to a person in a ring smaller than yours, someone closer to the center of the crisis, the goal is to help. Listening is often more helpful than talking. But if you're going to open your mouth, ask yourself if

what you are about to say is likely to provide comfort and support. If it isn't, don't say it.

"Don't, for example, give advice. People who are suffering from trauma don't need advice. They need comfort and support. So say, 'I'm sorry' or 'This must really be hard for you' or 'Can I bring you a pot roast?'

"Don't say, 'You should hear what happened to me' or 'Here's what I would do if I were you.' And don't say, 'This is really bringing me down.'

"If you want to scream or cry or complain, if you want to tell someone how shocked you are or how icky you feel, or whine about how it reminds you of all the terrible things that have happened to you lately, that's fine. It's a perfectly normal response. Just do it to someone in a bigger ring.

"Comfort IN, dump OUT."

I wish I had read this when we first started out, but this "ring theory" has been invaluable since. I never complained to Celeste but venting to my husband was totally fair game. Most people get this intrinsically, but you may meet or know a few people who could use this reminder.

So go ahead and find someone you trust who is a step or two away from the centre of the action. (Obviously today your child is in the centre ring and you are in one of the closest rings). Find a person who is out and complain away, and do a bit of emotional dumping. You'll need that release; it's a stressful time. To release stress, express.

Another way to release is to do something physical or creative. Go for a walk or a run. If your schedule allows, plan at least a little bit of exercise. It may not always be possible. My running came to a halt when we spent months in Toronto at Sick Kids, so instead I got creative.

What happened next became a story unto itself and opened up a new very healing world to me.

During chemo, Celeste's stepmom, Michelle, and I would take turns spending the night with Celeste. We would alternate twenty-four hours on and twenty-four hours off, swapping places just after lunchtime each day. When Michelle would arrive at the hospital, I would head back to Ronald McDonald House to eat dinner, do laundry, and rest.

These evenings were long and boring and gave me too much time on my own to think about Celeste. I don't normally watch TV and after a few bad experiences staying up to watch *Hoarders* and *Storage Wars* for too many hours, I realized I needed something to occupy my time so I wouldn't go crazy.

Downstairs, the house had a craft room for activities for the children staying at RMH. I asked the staff if I could use the craft room late at night when everyone was asleep. They said, "I don't see why not!"

I stopped by the dollar store on the way back from the hospital to pick up paints and canvasses, and then, at eleven o'clock at night, I laid my canvasses out on the craft table and started painting.

I love to paint acrylic abstract impressionism and that night I painted six paintings. When I was done, I gingerly carried them, one by one, up to my room to dry. I photographed them with my cell phone camera and the next day showed them off to Celeste.

"Look what Mummy did last night!"

It felt so good to do something creative and something just for me. It had been years since I had had an opportunity to paint with four children at home and no real craft/office space to use for my projects.

I decided to post the photos on my Facebook page and rename it Laura Lane, Author, Poet, and Artist. At my next opportunity to go home on the bus to my husband Matt, I packaged the paintings all up and took them with me.

Matt loved my paintings and asked if the next time I could paint using particular colours that he liked: red, black, silver, and gold. I agreed, but I had never done that before, having someone else suggest colours for me to use.

I took four canvasses and painted each a different background colour, then started layering and creating each canvas as I felt inspired by the colours. It worked wonderfully.

The next day when I was showing off my new paintings to Celeste, I suggested she choose four colours and I would create more paintings based on those colours. She chose blue, green, purple, and silver.

At my next opportunity in the craft room, I did another series of paintings. Celeste loved them. I then emailed Laurie and Hayley to tell them what I had been doing on my nights off and asked Hayley to choose four colours as well. Her colors were purple, pink, blue, and yellow.

I emailed the photos once I completed her paintings. Hayley's favorite she named *Waves* and it became my signature piece and my favorite too. It is the painting that has been incorporated onto the cover of this book.

It was such a blessing to me to be creative on my nights at Ronald McDonald House and it was thrilling to hear others people's positive feedback. One day the staff at RMH had come into my room for a regular safety inspection and were so surprised to find my little exhibit of paintings propped up all around the room.

I completed twenty-four paintings in those three months. I didn't quite know what to do with them. I had recently visited the Art Gallery of Ontario and viewed their contemporary art exhibit. An idea welled up within me. Maybe I could exhibit the paintings and tell people about Celeste and Hayley.

I wanted to express the story of our girls—the miracles we were experiencing—and tell about the power of prayer. I had all the paintings professionally photographed then set about finding galleries who were interested in showing the exhibit. I named the exhibit *Two Girls, One Prayer*.

I also decided I would auction off the paintings to raise money for Ronald McDonald House and Sick Kids Hospital in Toronto and to help with Hayley's medical bills.

I met an artist and curator at the QB Gallery in Thorold who was willing to exhibit the paintings. Soon enough, the paintings were framed and hung on the gallery walls. Local journalists interviewed me and took my picture. I was showing my work and telling the world about Celeste and Hayley.

The exhibit opening was December 2011. Other galleries agreed to have the exhibit in January and February. The February date was for the grand opening of a new gallery owned by the artist who had illustrated my children's book that I had released the previous summer. We had known each other for a number of years and I felt I knew her and trusted her.

Five days after the opening, this artist was arrested in the middle of the night for setting fire to her own gallery. All of my paintings and her life's work were lost in the fire. I was devastated. She was sentenced to prison for arson. There is no way of knowing or understanding why she did what she did. It was a tough setback.

We had found a creative outlet for expressing and it was healing. The girls were excited about the art gallery exhibits. To have that literally go up in flames was quite a blow.

Right after the fire, I attended an event Bob Proctor was hosting in Toronto. To be surrounded by positive creative people who encouraged me to look for the silver lining and pick up the pieces and move on was truly inspirational. By the end of the day, I was determined to have prints made of the paintings that were lost in the fire. I would create more paintings and put a call out to other artists to donate pieces to the art auction.

My auction would now be bigger and better than I originally planned.

Expression comes in different ways. I have asked for some of the ashes of the art gallery fire so that they can be used to create a special piece of art, just like a phoenix being born out of the ashes.

I continue to express with my art and continue to rebuild my life. I have now opened my own office, studio, and gallery. Creating abstract paintings with four colours has become my signature style. It has remained a creative outlet for me. It was and continues to be an emotional lifesaver for me.

I highly recommend everyone find some sort of creative outlet, some way to express. Just as you need to express your feelings by talking with a trusted someone, you need to express nonverbally too.

You never know where the expressing of yourself will lead you. Being courageous enough to be vulnerable, to open our hearts up, can lead us to deeper relationships with God, friends, and family, and it can provide peace. You may even find you love it! Which leads me to my last point, LOVE!

"It is good to love many things, for therein lies the true strength, and whosoever loves much performs much, and can accomplish much, and what is done in love is well done."

VINCENT VAN GOGH

Chapter 11

LOVE

Parenting is one of the hardest jobs you'll ever have to do. Once you learn that your child has cancer, your job becomes ten times more difficult.

Along with the normal parenting stresses, now you don't know if your child will live or die. Your whole life gets uprooted. You now have to care for your child; deal with hospitals, appointments, diagnosis, medications; and perhaps even move to another city or endure long commutes to the hospital.

It can be exhausting. But you do it. Of course, you do it. Sometimes in a haze, sometimes in joy, sometimes in fear. But you do it.

If you have other children at home, as most of us do, parenting them or even spending time with them will be more difficult. They still need you and you need them. But the cancer always seems to be there, taking priority over everything.

You may incur financial hardship. The stress may cause a huge strain on your marriage. You may experience depression or loneliness. You may have thoughts of "What could I have done differently?" The list goes on and on.

This is a time when you are going to need all the love you and your child can get.

French philosopher Yann Dall'Aglio's definition of love speaks to me: "Love is an expression of tenderness." To me, tenderness is about recognizing that something or someone is fragile. It is about being able to hold or embrace them in a manner that understands and accepts that if you treat them too roughly, they could break—physically or emotionally.

We are more readily able to accept the fragility of children and treat them tenderly, with great love and affection, eager to protect them from the world. When a child develops cancer, we are even more aware of their fragility and it becomes an opportunity to pour out our love on that child.

I cherish the moments I had when I could hold Celeste, cuddle her, sing to her, and love her. It was indeed a very tender time. During Celeste's first round of chemo and her transfer from a regular room to her isolation, no, her *healing* room, as her blood counts dropped, we were discouraged from contaminating her bed with germs. That's hard for a parent to hear: Don't sit on your sick child's bed.

But that didn't last long and I was climbing onto her bed again, holding and cuddling as much as possible. It was healing for both of us.

Love is a powerful emotion. It has the ability to create physiological changes in the body.

Love and hope and positive thoughts all have the ability to alter the body's neurochemistry. Dr. Jerome Groopman in *The Anatomy of Hope* explains how belief and expectation are able to "block pain by releasing the brain's endorphins and enkephalins, thereby mimicking the effects of morphine."

He goes on to explain in detail the substantiating research of the Benedetti experiment performed by Dr. Fabrizio Benedetti at the University of Turin in Italy. Numerous studies since the 1970s have established the link between love and the release of endorphins. From the research of Candace Pert and Nancy Ostrowski in 1976, psychiatrist Michael Liebowitz in 1983, and physician Theresa Crenshaw in 1996, there is evidence that love is more than just a warm fuzzy.

But any mother can tell you that: the fastest way to ease the pain of your child is to love and hold that child.

What is the first thing we do when our child falls down and scrapes her knee? We pick her up, hug and kiss her, and then apply the bandage. Love makes it "all better."

When Celeste was diagnosed, she was showered with love and affection. When we renamed her isolation room her *healing* room, I wrote all over the sliding glass door the names of all her friends and family who were loving and supporting her from a distance. Even though they couldn't come visit, I wanted her to know she was constantly surrounded with love. It was the same idea with the sticky notes right after her first surgery. I never wanted her to doubt how much she was loved. It became one of my biggest priorities.

Loving your child comes easily to most parents. Most of us don't need a reminder; we're doing it naturally. However, many mothers forget how to love themselves.

That is where I really like Yann Dall'Aglio's reminder that love is about tenderness. If we can begin to recognize our own fragility during this stressful time, we can be loving, kind, and patient with ourselves, our spouses, and our other children.

The diagnosis and treatment of cancer is a difficult situation for everyone. Stress is at an all-time high. This is when we need the greatest amounts of love, patience, and gratitude. This is where our true strength and character need to shine through.

Leo Buscaglia, the author of *Love* and the professor of Love 101 at University of Southern California, makes the observation that "Love requires one to be strong." He shares that "It is always from strength that gentleness arises," from our courage to be willing to be vulnerable.

I learned a great deal about love reading Og Mandino's book *The Greatest Salesman in the World* and the second scroll, which reminds us of the miracles and blessings that come when we are willing to say "I will greet this day with love in my heart."

Sometimes it is not easy to do that when we are tired and our child is sick.

Dave Blanchard, in his book *Today I Begin a New Life*, analyzes that wisdom by explaining the different forms of love. The word *charity* that we use today comes from the Greek word *agape*, which means "a heightened level of awareness." I have heard Blanchard explain further that it is "to see someone as God sees them."

When we can see everyone the way God sees them, all their frailties and weaknesses as well as their strengths, we can learn to treat them tenderly. We must also view ourselves from God's perspective: lovingly, tenderly, and patiently. We can do the same with our spouses and other children or family members.

Charity is also known as the pure love of Christ. It is how Jesus Christ saw and treated everyone. He saw them as God saw them and treated them with the utmost respect, love, and tenderness. The apostle Paul in the New Testament in the Bible explains that charity "beareth all things, believeth all things, hopeth all things, endureth all things. 1 Corinthians 13:7 (KJV)

Charity is the third Pillar of Islam or zakat. In Judaism, it is referred to as Tzedakah. In Hinduism, Buddhism, and Jainism, it is similarly known as Dana, the practice of unattached and unconditional generosity.

That kind of love, or charity, heals and transforms.

When you love something or someone it transforms that thing or person. When you allow yourself to be loved, it transforms you. When we root ourselves so that we are experiencing love on all levels—feeling it in our body and heart, accepting love, surrounded by love, generating love—then we are giving as well as receiving at the same time that we are connected to God.

But we have to remember that we can't give something until we have fully received it. That is why it is so important to allow ourselves to be loved.

Now what does that really mean? First we have to understand that the moment we love someone, we are no longer judging that person; and the moment we are judging someone, we are no longer loving him or her. "If you judge people, you have no time to love them," Mother Teresa said.

Brené Brown does a great job explaining our own difficulties in accepting help and love, and it stems from our own self-judgment or lack of self-love. On "Oprah's Lifeclass," Brown spelled it out to the audience.

"When you cannot accept and ask for help without self-judgment, then when you offer other people help, you are always doing so with judgment. Because you have attached judgment to asking for help.

"When you extract worthiness for helping people, that's judgment. When you don't extract worthiness and you think, 'I'm just helping you because one day I'm gonna need help'—that's connection. That's vulnerability."

If you are having difficulty allowing others to help you during your hour of need, it may be because of the judgment you have placed on others when you have helped them or judgment about your own worthiness in receiving help.

Courageously pull down the wall called judgment and begin tenderly loving you and those around you.

In this stressful time, you need love. You need to accept love and support. Go back to what I shared earlier about Ho'oponopono. Have a silent conversation with God and say, "I'm sorry I have been stuck in a feeling of judgment. Please forgive me. Thank you. I love you!"

Keep saying it until you are finally filled with feelings of love and gratitude.

Gratitude is the final peace of the puzzle. It is so important to have gratitude and love and appreciation for all those people supporting you and your child at this time.

For all the doctors, wonderful nurses who are there day and night, the multitude of support staff, hospital staff, social workers, chaplains, clergy, church groups, friends, neighbours, and family who are there to help with everything, feel the gratitude deep within you.

It may be impossible to thank every one of them, but if you can feel that gratitude in your heart for all they do, remembering their sacrifices, it will make some days easier to bear.

There will be days when people make mistakes, but if you have an attitude of gratitude, a bigger perspective, you can be more forgiving and loving. Think of how much your child loves and is grateful for you and all you do. Begin to feel the same love and gratitude for those around you. Our children really are our teachers. Celeste has taught me.

I truly believe that the children who are diagnosed with cancer are some of the wisest, sweetest, strongest, and most loving children. They have gained a bigger perspective of the world in such a short time. They become wise beyond their years.

Another thing we can learn to do is to be more grateful for every day we have with our children. None of us ever knows how long we have on Earth, so it is imperative that we live and love each moment we have. For some of us, our children's days do become numbered and we learn how to make the best of every moment we have left with them.

One of the gifts of our experience was that we learned a deeper meaning of love, a deeper way to love. As a mom, I realized it was not my job to only give love, but to also receive it. To learn to love and accept myself without judgment was part of the process.

My readings, my interactions with so many loving people, my time in prayer, and certainly my daughter, taught me more about love than I ever could have witnessed prior to Celeste's getting cancer.

It may not come easily on some days to greet each day with love, but when you do, you will feel the reward. Love does make us feel better, from the inside out. You can read the studies, but the only research that matters is what you experience for yourself.

Love is an expression of tenderness. Practice it in all ways. Of course you will be tender and loving to your child. Express that same love to the rest of the family, your spouse, and, most importantly, yourself.

There is so much love around you. Let it in. Let it ease the burden. Let it envelope you and hold you ever so tenderly as you journey through these days.

No matter what happens, Love always stays.

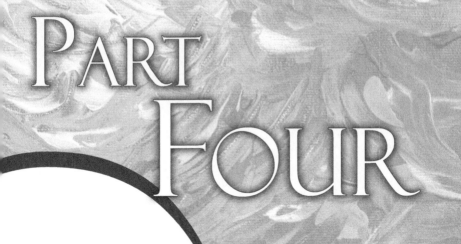

PART
FOUR

Chapter 12

HOW DO YOU COPE WHEN THE WORST HAPPENS?

This is the "difficult" chapter in other books that I never wanted to read. I was bound and determined that it wouldn't happen to my child. I was sorry that others had to lose their children, but it wasn't going to happen to me, to us, to Celeste.

If anyone could make a miracle happen, it was me. I believed in miracles, I saw miracles happen, and I had enough faith and determination to do everything in my power so my beautiful daughter would conquer these stupid cells in her body. I knew they were only cells in the wrong place, growing where they shouldn't, just a small task for Heavenly Father to take care of.

I knew we would have the miracle we were praying for.

I learned so much that year that I began teaching what faith really is all about: believing, listening, trusting, and acting. I believe in a God of miracles. I was willing to listen to the prompting I received from God, trust those promptings and act by following through on the inspiration I received. This wasn't hard. I was practicing my faith: believing, listening, trusting, and acting. I knew we could remain positive through it all and inspire others on how to bravely get through similar challenges.

What I didn't know was Heavenly Father's plan for Celeste.

We did receive miracles, so many miracles. Celeste's tumor shrank 98.5 percent; her cyst disappeared completely. She learned to walk again and run; she went back to school; she graduated grade eight with honours having missed four months of school; and she received the citizenship award and overall academic achievement award! She attended camp, acting classes, and youth leadership conference. She organized first her elementary school, then her high school participation in the Brain Tumour Foundation 5K Spring Sprint. She inspired thousands of people: family, friends, and strangers with her hope, strength, and courage. We were seeing miracles!

But in the summer of 2012, Celeste's June MRI showed some spots that hadn't been there before. Others had reported similar early MRIs showing new spots but they end up being nothing or were gone on the next MRI. We prayed that would be the case with Celeste. But in those first few days after hearing the news, I was overcome with fear of losing her.

What if? I couldn't bear the thought.

I rededicated myself to doing everything to help her return to full health. I prayed and focused on seeing her healthy and happy. I asked everyone we knew to refocus and keep praying for her full recovery. I studied Wayne Dyer's book *The Power of Intention*. I continued to ask my Heavenly Father and I was ready to receive answers, blessings, and miracles.

I was willing to do everything necessary to help Celeste. Although the medical system didn't have anything else left to offer, there were still many more options available alternatively. I knew prayer was the greatest tool we had. But I realized that ultimately it was up to Celeste and what she wanted.

It was her fight, not mine.

She's the one in the ring. It was her choice and not mine. If Celeste wanted to live, then I would help in every way possible. But if she didn't have the energy left to do this anymore, then I would support her in that as well.

We would focus on helping her to live the best way possible with the time she had remaining and make every day fantastic!

This was the hardest thing to do, but it was what gave me the most peace. It was the ultimate letting go.

No one wants to really believe they are going to lose their child. It was not the outcome we wanted. Two mothers, one prayer. One daughter lived. One did not. Not the "happy ending" that TV movies are made of.

If you want to skip this chapter, I understand. As I said, I didn't like to read these chapters. I can't tell you what to do, what to feel, or what decisions to make. I can only tell you our story and pray you can find a glimmer of hope, a truth that resonates or something that inspires you that you, too, can get through these dark days.

This chapter is about the last eight months of my daughter's life.

Yes, a small fraction of this part of the story is about hospitals and procedures and her declining health; truly, this chapter is about living life, about faith, and creating something beautiful in the moment and forever.

The summer of 2012 began with the end of school activities. The grade eight trip to Niagara Falls and Toronto, and then graduation. Celeste graduated with honors, the overall academic achievement award, and the citizenship award. We had a beautiful dress made especially for Celeste, made completely out of neckties, with a hat to match. She was happy and vibrant and we were so thrilled to see how well she was recovering. She was walking well and even beginning to run again too.

Earlier that spring, Celeste had participated in the Brain Tumour Foundation of Canada 5K Spring Sprint, walking the whole distance, and encouraging more than thirty students and staff to participate in a team together. Michelle and I, Connlan and Grayson, and our dear friend, Ginette, all walked alongside Celeste as she completed the walk using her cane for support.

Celeste had her next MRI at the end of June, but it would be weeks before we finally learned the results. In the meantime, the summer was planned and filled with fun activities and enjoying her improved health.

In July, Celeste and I went to Girls Camp, camping in tents, doing crafts, tubing on the lake, canoeing and enjoying campfire activities. Not much slowed her down; she participated in just about every activity and shared her testimony, her belief in God, setting an example for the girls around her.

She also had family time at a cottage with her grandma, aunts, and cousins. The summer also included things Celeste loved best— private acting classes, preparing monologues, and time in front of the camera, and then Youth Leadership Conference, meeting youth from all across southern Ontario.

I attended YLC with Celeste. She took part in as many activities as possible, especially enjoying the dances and meeting a special, kind, young man who danced and talked with her all evening. She made new friends and boldly answered questions, volunteering during workshops and fully participating in the physical and service activities.

It was a great summer and I felt privileged that she asked me to attend most of her activities with her: going on rides with her at Niagara Falls, sharing her tent at Girls Camp, rooming together at Leadership. I will be forever be grateful for all those memories and time spent together that summer.

I'm still not sure why we didn't hear back from the doctor sooner about the MRI results, but it wasn't until September that I finally learned about the newfound spots. We had simply assumed that no news meant good news.

One of Laurie's greatest fears had been waiting on Hayley's MRI results. What if they found something new? What if the cancer came back? I was the opposite, always so focused on receiving the much anticipated "No Evidence of Disease" (NED) that I wasn't worried at all. I always anticipated hearing more good news. I knew Celeste was going to continue to improve. Hearing the opposite was quite a shock.

My mind scrambled to cope and figure out what to hold on to, how to continue to remain positive.

It was that same week that Laurie attended a conference at the Children's Hospital of Philadelphia, meeting with doctors and parents about brain tumour research, protocols, etc. She informed me that many parents expressed that many times they would have MRI results come back with new spots and on the next MRI it would turn out to be nothing or completely gone. That is where I put all my hope.

Next it was time to tell Celeste. As we were driving to a church dance, I told her we finally had received the results of her MRI, and they found new spots and the doctors didn't have any treatment options for her. She had done her protocol, and that was that.

But I told her there were always other things that could be done. We have the power of prayer and energy treatments and we would learn about anything that was out there that could help.

I would do anything to help my daughter, and Celeste knew that. I had also come to the realization that this wasn't my fight and I told my darling daughter that if she wanted to live, to fight this, we would do everything we could to help her, but if she felt she just couldn't do this any more, if it was too hard and too much to ask, then we would do everything to make every day she has with us beautiful and fulfilling. Whether that was three months or three years, we would make it wonderful. It was up to her.

Celeste very boldly said she wanted to live and wanted to fight it.

I told her what Laurie said about spots sometimes turning out to be nothing and we would talk to her doctor and see what happened on the next MRI in October. So we left it at that.

Celeste had a great time at the dance—so strong and so brave and beautiful and trusting. I quietly pulled aside our wonderful priesthood leader to tell him the news. I wanted to be brave and strong and calm, and I still don't know how I even got the words out of my mouth. How do you tell someone that maybe, just maybe, your little girl wasn't going to make it?

I hadn't allowed myself to entertain that thought.

I clung to my faith, my hope, my vision of her being healed and carried on again. I clung to the normalcy of life. We went home, I cooked her favorite meals, and we did our regular family activities. I just prayed that everything would be OK.

I asked Celeste what she wanted me to tell people. I knew we needed the extra prayers again, but I didn't want people focusing on the worst, so we posted: "Hi Everyone! Celeste asked me to share with you that she is doing fantastic! We are so very grateful for all your constant prayers and support over the last eighteen months. Please keep visualizing and praying for her complete health. Here is the video we created last year to help with the visualization." http:// tinyurl.com/l39a95t

The day of the doctor's appointment in October, I sat with Celeste and her dad and the doctor. Without the doctor having any additional treatments to offer, Celeste's dad was not interested in any more MRIs. I insisted she had to have follow up, and he agreed that the usual one-year follow up MRI could be done next June.

We posted to our prayer warriors: "Today's wonderful update! Just back from Celeste's doctor appt. She's doing great! Next appointment is February and we are not worrying about MRIs until next June, one year from her last one! Yeah! Thank you everyone for your continued prayers and visualizing Celeste in complete health! We love and appreciate you for all your support through the last twenty months."

We carried on with life. Celeste had started high school in London and loved going to school with Desiree. They walked home from school together and Celeste would spend lunches with Desy as well. She was outgoing and participating in school activities. She was helping to organize a school team to participate in the Brain Tumour Foundation of Canada annual Spring Sprint. It would be her third year walking the 5K.

Celeste was easily recognized around school, boldly wearing her ties and sporting her white baseball cap or unabashedly being the girl with little to no hair. She was a member of the school spirit team helping with the morning video announcements. She was well loved by her teachers, who noticed her mature attitude. She wasn't like the other kids in that she didn't get caught up in petty issues. She had already learned that those sorts of things really weren't worth worrying about, not when you put things into perspective.

I worried about her. It didn't seem like she had the friends around that she had before. After school, she was tired and couldn't do sports and other after-school activities. She didn't have her own group of girl friends to hang out with at lunch or weekends. I talked with her about moving back home with me in Niagara. I knew that was where she really wanted to be and we talked about her moving between semesters or the end of the school year.

She had started experiencing some pains in her leg and was getting increasingly tired. I worried that high school was just too much for her. I knew Hayley was having similar struggles. They were still recovering from all that chemo and radiation. We knew it would be a while before they would be 100 percent back to normal.

As Christmas came along, the tiredness seemed to be getting worse. Celeste was looking forward to attending an overnight youth activity between Christmas and New Year's. She had attended last year and looked forward to being able to participate more this year. It proved to be a long and difficult outing.

We had arrived late and missed eating dinner with everyone. She didn't have the strength to stay up late after the movie when everyone else was running around in the snow. She just wanted to go to bed. We had been given a private room for just her and me rather than bunking in with a group of girls. That also meant she was not enjoying the slumber party fun happening in the dorm rooms either. She didn't know whom to sit with and the other girls didn't know how to include her. It was hard to watch.

I wanted her to have fun and enjoy her time there. In the morning, she again felt tired and we arrived late to breakfast. She attended a few workshops but she was not only tired but also now having headaches and double vision. This was not good. She went to lie down and I arranged for her to receive a blessing.

We called Michelle, who called the doctor, who recommended we make the two-hour drive to London immediately. Celeste was given a blessing and we loaded up our stuff in the car. She slept most of the way there. I had called Matt and he and the kids made their way to London as well. By the time we arrived at the emergency room, she had eaten half a sandwich and was feeling much better. The headaches were gone and so was the double vision.

The doctor looked her over and said if she had something more to eat he would let her go home. He prescribed medicine and she was even given permission to fly to Utah to visit family, but we should arrange an MRI after she got back.

I wrote a letter and posted it for our friends, family, and supporters:

> Happy New Year everyone! We are so very thankful for all the support our family has received throughout 2012. It was a long year and Celeste has done incredibly well. She has been feeling quite tired this last month and we are reminded of the necessity to redouble our efforts to keep Celeste in our prayers.
>
> This last weekend Celeste attended our local overnight youth activity but had to leave early to check in with doctors because of the symptoms she was having. A special prayer service was held for Celeste. All the youth and leaders held hands and created a special prayer circle on Celeste's behalf. The strong sense of love and support for Celeste was felt by the whole group and us. The timing of this prayer was a blessing to Celeste as it was said just as we arrived at the hospital. By the time the doctor arrived,

Celeste's headache and double vision had cleared up and she was alert and happy. The doctor sent her home once she could show that she was fine eating something, and she is allowed to travel to visit family in Utah and come to the clinic when she gets back.

Celeste has been such a trouper over the last two years but we have been reminded that she isn't completely out of the woods yet. It is such a long haul—a real marathon of a feat to overcome. This is an Olympic feat and, like any athlete who goes to the Olympics, they don't do it alone. They have a whole country behind them supporting them. Celeste needs to know now that she is not alone. (She feels very alone—so few people understand what exactly she is going through and find it hard to approach her at school or church.) She really needs to know we support her and love her and she needs our prayers more than ever as she is tiring from the effort she has put into healing these last two years. She needs to be reminded of how strong she is and how far she has come and we are supporting her to victory.

Celeste is such a beautiful, sweet spirit and she has been told on numerous occasions that she has a special work to do here in this life. Let's buoy her up so she can be and do everything she is meant to do in this life.

Please share this request for prayers with as many people and prayer circles as possible. Two years ago, Celeste had thousands of people praying for her all over the world. We need to do that again. Prayer is such a powerful tool. We saw what a huge difference it made in shrinking her tumours last time. Let's do it again to visualize Celeste in complete health now so she can live out a long and happy life.

If you are a friend of Celeste, now is the time to reach out to her and help her feel included and living a healthy, happy, vibrant life again.

With sincerest gratitude,

Celeste's mum,
Laura Lane

Let's make 2013 a year filled with hope, strength, and courage!

As you can see, that was my rally cry.

On January 1, Celeste, Desy, and Connlan flew to Utah with their dad and Michelle. They had a great trip visiting all their grandparents, aunts, uncles, and more than twenty cousins. She was fussed over a lot, which drove her crazy, but still she had a great time. They flew back on January 8 and the MRI was scheduled for Friday, January 11.

There is no way we could be prepared for the news we were about to receive that day.

I sat next to Celeste, sitting in the rocking chair with earplugs in my ears, reading and making notes in my journal, while she had her MRI. From there we went to another floor for her bone scan. It was a cold room and we both had blankets to keep us warm. Michelle texted me. The results from the MRI didn't look good.

Michelle had stayed behind in radiology to see if she could use her contacts to find out more before we met with the doctors.

While Celeste lay on the scanner, I asked if she could do anything in the world, what would she like to do?

Top of the list: Travel to London, England, to see Big Ben, and then travel to Paris, France, and visit the Eiffel Tower and eat real pain au chocolat. And she wanted Hayley to come with us. She wanted to visit Switzerland and travel first class! She wanted to go to Italy and see the Leaning Tower of Pisa.

I asked her if she could meet anyone in the whole world whom would she like to meet? Robin Williams and Anne Hathaway, the cast of *Doctor Who* and Celine Dion.

We went on to make a wonderful bucket list including things like going to the Mandarin Restaurant, trying new foods, spa treatments, climbing a rock wall, making homemade Nanaimo bars, having reunion parties with the cast of *To Kill a Mockingbird* and her French immersion class, and receiving her patriarchal blessing.

She wanted Hayley to come to Grandad's Soup Party in February to meet my Godmother Aunty Jill and her family. We ended up making a list of forty-seven things.

After the scan was done, we had enough time to go for lunch in the hospital bistro lunchroom before meeting the doctors to find out the results. Celeste was all about trying new foods. She and I shared two sandwiches and three types of soup. I took photos of her beautiful smiling face as she showed off her discoveries of new foods she liked.

Then it was time to meet with the doctor. The results were much worse than anyone expected. There were tumours all over her brain.

There was evidence of a recent bleed, probably the day we had raced to the ER from the youth activity, but it had miraculously stopped. (I know that was the blessing of the group prayer that afternoon.)

We asked what does that mean? How much time does she have left?

The doctor explained that with the amount of cancer in her body she might only live a few days or weeks, but they didn't expect her to last the month.

How could it be that my little girl had only days or weeks?

I was stunned but at the same time peaceful. I was prepared for this. I had already decided what I was going to do. We had already started. We would make every day she had with us wonderful.

Celeste was supposed to come home with me that afternoon but the doctors didn't want her to travel until her meds were stabilized. I called Matt and told him to pack bags and bring Grayson. We would need to stay in London.

We booked in at a hotel with a waterslide in hopes of having some fun with the children. It was Connlan's birthday that weekend. The first thing we did was play a *Doctor Who* Monopoly game together, then we all went out to the Mandarin restaurant for dinner. It was the first time all eight of us, the four kids plus me and Matt, and my ex and Michelle, had ever sat down to eat together.

Celeste tried a bunch of new foods, including crab and lobster. We went back to her dad's house and stayed until Celeste fell asleep. She wanted me to stay the night but I knew I needed to be with Matt that night. I knew I was going to need someone to hold me while I cried.

Celeste slept all day Saturday until 5:00 p.m. When I went over again later, the church had already started sending meals over. They did so for the next six weeks. That night I did stay the night, sleeping on a mattress on the floor of Celeste's room. It was our slumber party. Desy and I cuddled with Celeste until she fell asleep.

Sunday morning Celeste and I went to church. Grandma Sharon, Uncle Rick, and Aunty Crystal drove in from Hamilton to be with us. We had arranged for her patriarchal blessing. This is a very special blessing that is only given once in a person's lifetime and it usually gives the recipient guidance from the Lord about the individual's talents and blessings needed to help with future decisions in living life.

The patriarch had made a special trip into London just for Celeste. Bishop Baxter and I sat with Celeste as she received her blessing. It was beautiful. After it was done, all five of us—Celeste and I, Sharon, Rick, and Crystal—sat together with the bishop to discuss the Lord's words to Celeste. She had been told what to expect as she made her transition, that she would be taken to her Heavenly Father and the Saviour and she would be enveloped in love and gratitude and she would be greeted by angels and family.

She was blessed to know that she had gained eternal life and would rise in the morning of the first resurrection. Her calling and election has been made sure. Bishop Baxter shared how humbled he was to hear such a pronouncement made. It was something we all strive for and to know she had been given that blessing and knowledge truly took the sting out of death. She was told how very special she was. It was a beautiful experience.

Celeste went to join the other young women for Sunday school and I stayed to talk to the bishop about planning a memorial service. We were going to have the funeral at the chapel near my house in Niagara but wanted a second memorial service here in London.

That night we celebrated Connlan's birthday and I settled in for another night sleeping on the floor of Celeste's room. I was waiting for the news that Celeste was safe to drive the two hours home to our house. In the mean time, we began posting on Facebook and emailing and working on granting Celeste's final wishes.

This is some of what we posted:

From Matt:

Some of you know of my daughter Celeste and the battle she's had the past couple of years with cancer. I am pained to have to inform you that the cancer has returned and at a much larger scale than her original prognosis from two years ago. Celeste has numerous tumours throughout her brain and spinal column. The doctors are not expecting her to last another month.

Our family is now using this time to spend with Celeste to make her as comfortable as possible. Celeste has chosen to end her days at home and not in the hospital; for now that is in London with her father, stepmother and siblings, but we hope to get her home in Fonthill to do some other things she wants.

I would like to thank all of our friends for the support you have shown over the last couple of years. It really means a lot to our family to have the support we have received from all of you. Thank you.

From me:

Thank you everyone for your outpouring of love and support right now. For anyone who doesn't know yet, Celeste had her MRI and bone scan. Her cancer has spread all over her brain and spine. Her doctor has said with this amount of disease in her body she could last days or weeks, but may not last the month.

Celeste is aware of her situation and is still such a strong girl, participating in conversations about her final wishes. We have made a wish list of things she would like to do, which include some parties with friends, making Nanaimo bars with the YW in London, climbing to the top of a rock climbing wall, and meeting Robin Williams, Anne Hathaway, Celine Dion, and the cast of *Doctor Who*.

This is where we could use everyone's help. If you know anyone who knows anyone in the TV, film, or music industry who can expedite this request for us, it would be greatly appreciated.

Thank you for all your messages of support. I do read them all but am not able to respond to everyone right now, but thank you very much!

It's amazing what can happen when you ask! The doctors said she couldn't travel to Europe so we put all our focus on having some parties and getting hold of celebrities. Within four days of writing her list, she had her first surprise phone call. Then every day got better and better. Within seven days she had spoken to four celebrities. I shared our thanks:

15 January: Some totally awesome person worked our first wish miracle: Celeste just received a call from David Tenant! That was so cool and a total surprise!

16 January: Woohoo! Celeste just had a fourteen-minute Skype call with Robin Williams! He's going to call her again in a few days when he is home from touring so he can show her his pets and view of the ocean in San Francisco! Thank you to everyone who made this possible.

HOW DO YOU COPE WHEN THE WORST HAPPENS?

Hollywood has been bombarded with requests to make this happen.

17 January: We have one very special lucky girl! This evening Celeste received a call from Celine Dion! She sent Celeste her love and told her how special she is. She took time out of her very busy schedule to talk to Celeste right before her show. We are so very grateful to everyone who worked hard to make this happen and thankful to Celine Dion for bringing more happiness to Celeste as well.

18 January: This was the coolest ever! Anne Hathaway Skyped with Celeste for forty minutes! They just became new best friends! Anne wants make sure that this was only an introduction and they will talk as much as possible. They talked about Celeste's tie dress, their favourite books and movies and pets. She introduced us to her husband and dog. She even sang Queen's "Somebody to Love" that she had sung in *Ella Enchanted*. It was so cool! Thank you to everyone who made this possible, especially Kelly and her friend Johanna.

21 January: We were able to grant a few more wishes for Celeste this weekend. Friday night included dinner at her favourite restaurant, MacRoni's in Hamilton, and she enjoyed trying a number of pasta dishes she hadn't tried before. She said the lasagne was delicious.

Saturday was a wonderful day. Hayley and her parents arrived from New Jersey and Grandad hosted his famous soup party at Celeste's request to have it a month early this year. Celeste loved Joanna's Lobster Bisque; she ate three bowls! She also stole my bowl of Grandad's oxtail soup—one of my favorites—and she tried a number of other soups as well. It was wonderful to see so many friends and family members out this year.

One of Celeste's other wishes was to be in a movie, so we arranged for Ed Limon and Phoenix Gate Pictures Video production team to come out and film a mini documentary about Celeste and Hayley. Thanks also to Alex Sears for photographing the day for us. We'll share photos with everyone soon.

Sunday was a more difficult day for Celeste with some pain in her legs in the morning but after a priesthood blessing she was able to better enjoy the rest of the day at Grandma Sharon's house.

Celeste felt well enough to post on Facebook as well!

22 January: Don't just talk about the soup, Mummy! You need to be getting the recipes so I can eat more of it. What did you do with the stuff Grandad gave us at the end of the night of what was left of the oxtail soup anyway?

Michelle joined in too: The Celeste-bration was a great success! Celeste had lots of fun visiting with friends and family. Thank you to everyone who helped in the planning, and to everyone who came to make our girl's night brighter!

We kept the excitement going.

23 January: Celeste received a special package from Celine Dion: an autographed photo and she has another

package from California waiting to be picked up from FedEx! Can't wait to find out what is arriving from L.A.!

23 January: Drum roll! Celeste just received a package from Jim Carrey!! She received a signed box set of six movies! *Yes Man, Liar Liar, Mr Popper's Penguins, Dumb and Dumber, Mask,* and *The Truman Show*! Totally awesome and thoughtful of Jim to send this along to Celeste!

25 January: Another big THANK YOU to Robin Williams for taking the time again yesterday to Skype with Celeste. He introduced her to his cute dog Leonard and his cat as well! He was kind enough to take time in his busy schedule before flying off to do a show in L.A. Celeste had a good day, which included a short visit with Grandad and plans to watch more Jim Carrey movies!

25 January: Totally cool! Celeste just received a video message from Karen Gillan, "Amy" in the last few seasons of *Doctor Who*! That was so nice of her! Celeste loved it and was totally surprised and very thankful—it came at the right time to lift her spirits tonight. Thank you!

26 January: Celeste received a beautiful gift from singer/songwriter/musician Fiz. He created a beautiful song for Celeste that we have created a special video to go with it. http://tinyurl.com/ls8sx7q

26 January: Fiz De Mattia, if I may. I met Laura at a Bob Proctor event recently. We normally speak every week as she is in my Mastermind Group. Laura shared with our group that Celeste needed prayers. I felt like I needed to write a healing song to help Celeste. This took priority

over my life, but I was having a hard time writing it. I knew something was up but I didn't quite know what. Well, about a week later Laura shared that the doctors said there wasn't much time. Then I knew why I had a hard time with the healing song. I was supposed to write a different song, a song to help Celeste on her journey. The divine helped me write this, as they are waiting for this angel. I ask that you sing this song to help Celeste with a beautiful, smooth transition. That is the reason for this song. The title is called "Angel on a Stage" because Celeste wanted to be an actress. "The Lord is waiting there for you, he knows your heart is pure and true."

As you can see, our prayers were being answered now, in a different way. We were showering Celeste with so much love and support. It was a different kind of healing.

On February 6, the staff of OWN Life Story Project mailed us a copy of their "Loyalty and Betrayal" episode that was airing that night so that Celeste could watch it. Celeste and I had been interviewed in June of the previous year, sharing our story of friendship with Hayley and Laurie. She was now officially a TV star too!

We were able to keep fulfilling Celeste's bucket list. From a manicure/pedicure outing with Michelle, Grandma Heather, Desy, and Mummy, to another long Skype chat with Anne Hathaway and a twenty-minute call from Matt Smith (the newest doctor in the *Doctor Who* series) in London, England, to time spent with Matt and Grayson.

We were so very grateful for all those who helped make it all happen. This huge outpouring of love, day after day after day, was such a blessing to all of us. Knowing that people cared so much to do these things for my little girl meant the world to me. Watching the happiness it brought to Celeste was amazing. Making sure she knew how very special she was mattered more to me than anything else. That it was inspiring others at the same time was icing on the cake.

We received messages from friends sharing how friends of friends of friends were all sharing Celeste's story. Word kept coming back to us how it was inspiring hundreds and maybe thousands of people.

During those last weeks, it became important again to let people know what exactly we were hoping and praying for Celeste. It was also an opportunity to share the understanding and peace I had received during this difficult time. I posted this note to Facebook on January 31:

> Thank you, everyone, for all your prayers and support. Many have been asking how Celeste is doing. A number of people have also been sending various types of kind suggestions to help Celeste heal and praying for a miracle. I'd like to ask for your prayers and fasting for this Sunday, but I want to explain about what exactly we would like you to specifically pray for on Celeste's behalf.

> During the last three weeks since we received the diagnosis of just how much cancer has spread through her young body and how long she is expected to endure that amount of disease, I have come to understand the bigger picture as to why my little girl needs to go home to her Heavenly Father and why it is not only the best thing for her but a beautiful gift.

> A member of our clergy shared with our congregation at home that sometimes there are spirits that are so precious and so sweet and innocent and special that our Heavenly

Father has to bring them home. I want to share with anyone who doesn't know Celeste well, that she is one of
those sweet precious spirits, and anyone who knows Celeste well can tell you that yes she is indeed a very special
young lady. Celeste is so sensitive to everything and everyone around her. I believe that her Heavenly Father has
looked down at her and said, "My precious little girl, you
don't need to stay in this world any longer, I am bringing
you home now." This a blessing to Celeste. To keep her in
this world would be cruel. She needs to go home to her
Heavenly Father's embrace.

There can still be miracles in her return to her Heavenly
home. I do not believe that she has to suffer and die slowly to make her transition to the other side. I believe that
Heavenly Father can call her home at any time without
having to wait until her body shuts down from disease.
The doctors and nurses have shared their experiences with
this disease and how difficult it can be, but I know with
God nothing is impossible.

It is Celeste's desire to go peacefully in her sleep. That is
the miracle I would like you to pray and fast for on her
behalf. That is her last wish: That she can make a beautiful and peaceful transition without having to suffer pain
and discomfort.

She has done all she needs to do and has fought the good
fight and now it is time for her to rest in her Heavenly
Father's arms. She has been given a blessing that prepared
her for her transition and knows that she will be surrounded by angels who will take her back to her Heavenly

Father and she will be reunited with our family members who have gone on before us.

She is my little angel and I know she will become my new guardian angel and will be watching over me and our whole family for many years to come. It will be a great blessing to us to have her there helping us from the other side. She has and continues to inspire so many people around the world. I hope her precious spirit and strength and the comfort and peace we have at this time, understanding her call to go home, will continue to inspire you and give you peace and comfort now as well.

Celeste and I had many conversations in her final six weeks. I let her know that my mother and sister would be there to greet her as she made her transition.

When I was 9 years old, my mother and my 7-year-old sister and I had been in a tragic car accident that had killed both my mother and my sister. I literally walked away with only a cut on my finger. I knew I had been divinely protected. Over the years I had felt their presence in my life. I knew where they were and that they were watching over me. I would tease Celeste that now it would be her job to watch over me and keep me out of trouble.

One day as we were talking, she expressed how she was going to miss me. With tears in my eyes, I told her I was going to miss her too but she needed to understand something. I told her that everything I learned about being a mother I learned from my mother. Nana Joy passed away at the age of 38. That's just a few years younger than I was and not only that, but I looked just like my mother and sounded just like my mother.

Celeste would literally be going from one mother to another who would look and sound so much the same. This beautiful thought was also a comfort to me, knowing my precious little girl would be in the best hands. Over the years, many times I had felt my mother near me. I could usually tell it was her because I could feel her hands on my shoulders. Celeste and I made a pact that she would find a way to let me know that she was near by as well. Since her passing I have felt her close by many times and I have felt her rubbing my back in comfort.

There was another day that Celeste was having a hard time and lamenting the fact that the treatments she had undergone had slowed her growth. She hadn't fully gone through puberty yet. I shared with her another insight that I had, knowledge of a beautiful promise mothers have about their children.

When we come to this earth, we come to obtain a body, not an infant's body, not a child's body but a fully-grown adult body. That is part of God's plan for us. He has given us a promise that after the Saviour returns in his glory, there will be 1,000 years of peace on the earth—the Millennium. During that time, the righteous mothers will have the opportunity to return to earth and raise their children.

I already knew that one day my mother would get to come back and raise my sister—she was only 7 when she died. Now I have the promise that I can come back to raise Celeste until she is fully-grown as well. Every mother that has lost a child has that promise. And what a blessing that will be to do so during a time of peace on earth. There will be no lost opportunities; we just get to do it later. I can really see how Heavenly Father knew what would be best for Celeste. She gets to come back later when the world is a much more beautiful place to live in.

We are big fans of *Doctor Who*, so I compared what we were doing with an episode called "The Girl in the Fireplace." In the story, the Doctor keeps popping into Madame De Pompadour's life at different points. She begins to notice that, for him, it's only minutes that have gone by, but for her years have passed. She knows she will meet him again but she must take the slow path while he jumps ahead.

It will be like that for Celeste and me. I must take the slow path through life, and for her when we meet again it might only feel like moments have passed. This is the glorious hope, the beautiful vision that I have and that keeps me going. These were the things we shared and talked about in the little time we had left together.

In Celeste's last week or two, she began to ask me where the music was coming from. She would be sitting in the kitchen or in her room. She could hear the angelic choirs. Or she would ask me who it was that was sitting on the end of her bed? I could only respond that I was sure it was someone really nice but I couldn't see who it was myself.

I am so thankful that she was having these experiences and that she was sharing them with me. While I couldn't see the angels, I could definitely feel their presence around me. They were not only supporting her, they were also holding me together emotionally, too. I knew it had a great deal to do with all the prayers that were being said for our family at this time. We had earth angels helping us too. We were being supported in so many ways.

When it was no longer feasible for me to sleep on the floor in Celeste's room, when she had to be moved to the living room with a full hospital bed to accommodate her, I went to stay with a beautiful widow, Judy. She was from our church in London and she had a room for me (and Matt) to stay in and a room for Grayson as well. We had never met before but she opened her home to us and we became very close over those four weeks that I stayed with her.

Back home, many people were serving and helping us as well. Our neighbor, Trish, made sure our driveway and walks were always clear. Every time it snowed in those six weeks, she was out there with her snow blower. Matt's boss, Mark, made it possible for Matt to leave at any given notice, covering his shifts for him.

When we still hoped Celeste would make it home, our friends Sharon, Lina, and Claudia came over and painted the girls' room especially for her in blue and purple and a Winnie the Pooh bear theme. The young women from church came over and did a "heart attack," covering the room in hearts and love notes. Celeste was able to view their beautiful handiwork via Skype. Friends in London did the same thing to her room there, too. Celeste's friend Hannah even took care of our hamster. So many little things that meant the world to us.

Celeste was so very ready to make her transition. She wanted to go peacefully in her sleep. Each night she would wonder if this would be the night. The next morning she would wake up and complain with a pout that she didn't get to go yet.

She shared her wishes for her funeral and memorial services. We talked about who would speak and what songs she liked and that she wanted Nanaimo bars served. She chose the white dress she wanted to be buried in. We special ordered it and she saw it before she passed. She wanted her Pooh bear collection and stuffies to be shared among all her cousins. She was working on completing different pearler bead crafts for each family member as well.

Celeste kept amazing the nurses and doctors. One nurse didn't expect Celeste to still be with us when she came back from vacation but she was up eating ice cream and cake in the kitchen almost to the end. We let her eat anything she wanted. Many times that was cake for breakfast! One night she wanted to know if she had to brush her teeth? We certainly didn't have to worry about her teeth rotting. The only reason I could think of was that her breath might start to smell and we wouldn't want to kiss her. So she agreed to brush, but we weren't sticklers about it.

In the end, those last few days, she progressed quite quickly through those final stages, and we made sure she had as much morphine as she needed to be comfy. She began sleeping most of the day. Saturday evening she woke up and wanted to talk to her brothers and sister. She was completely lucid then went back to sleep. She had said her goodbyes to all our family. She was ready to make her transition.

Matt and I had stayed by her side that last night, pressing the button for her meds every twenty minutes all night. When the nurse arrived in the morning she let us know it would be soon.

She passed away just a few minutes before noon on Sunday, February 24, 2013.

Chapter 13

HOPE, STRENGTH, AND COURAGE

No matter your circumstance, there is hope, strength, and courage to be found.

There can be beauty and peace in helping your child make a graceful transition to heaven. There are miracles everywhere and can be found in every circumstance. Look for them.

There can be beauty and peace in helping your child make a graceful transition to "normal life." We are still two mothers, one prayer, and that is for the love and blessing of our daughters. Celeste is in Heaven; Hayley is still here on Earth.

We feel the love, always.

Miracles come from love. Miracles come from a seed of hope, a glimpse, a vision of something beautiful that makes our heart sing, something we can fall in love with so much that we are willing to trust and listen to inspiration. We can act on what we have been guided or led to do. That is when miracles happen; that is faith.

Take these little seeds of hope, grow them in your heart, love them, cherish them, and feed them until your vision engulfs you. We hope you find that this book is filled with little seeds of hope that you can plant in your heart, the birthing place of your own personal miracles.

We hope that you can find the needed strength to help your child fight this battle. That needed reservoir of strength is fed by our love for our children and it is contagious. You can gain strength from others' examples and by having hope and determination. Strength comes from will power, never giving up and a firm resolve.

Write these quotations in your journal or post them where you will see them.

"Strength does not come from physical capacity. It comes from an indomitable will."

Mahatma Gandhi

"Anyone can give up, it's the easiest thing in the world to do. But to hold it together when everyone else would understand if you fell apart, that's true strength."

Unknown

"When you come to the end of your rope, tie a knot and hang on."

Franklin D. Roosevelt

"I have learned over the years that when one's mind is made up, this diminishes fear."

Rosa Parks

We hope you will find a way to courageously allow others to be a part of your and your child's journey by sharing your heart and sharing your deep felt emotions and struggles with your family, friends, support people, and God. When you do, you will find the blessings of connection, acceptance, and love. Be brave for your child, hold on, and don't give up. Your child will appreciate you more than you can ever imagine.

Caroline Bailey in her blog Barren to Blessed writes:

> "Dear Parent of a Sick Child, what you are doing matters. Your strength, your wisdom, your love, your hope, your courage, and your presence are the greatest gifts you can give your child. Don't forget that, and don't be discouraged.
>
> ***Your child will remember your presence more than the pain.***"

That quotation sums up everything I want to share. I wouldn't give up a minute of the two years I spent with Celeste while she was sick. Every moment I spent holding her, cuddling in her bed until she fell asleep. All those nights, wide awake at 3:00 a.m. watching her sleep between nurse visits. Getting her up to pee every two hours on those chemo days. Or watching eight straight hours of *iCarly* because she wanted me to see every episode.

I wouldn't give away a single time of holding the bucket and cloth as she threw up for the twentieth time that day or helping her to the commode when I was so tired I could hardly see. Or writing Facebook posts asking for someone to bring me food because I couldn't even get away for five minutes to get something to eat in the cafeteria.

I loved that she needed and wanted me there. I couldn't take away her pain but I could hold her and love her and kiss her. I could tell the world how awesome she was. I could fill her room with well wishes from around the world so she would know she wasn't alone. I could convince the hospital staff that it was in her best interest to have special visitors like our clergy or my First Nation healer friend or her elementary school counselor or the missionaries to give her a blessing. I could make roast beef, Yorkshire pudding, and mashed potatoes or chicken couscous or any other food she wanted at the drop of a hat no matter who I had to call to have access to a kitchen in downtown Toronto.

I read every book necessary to develop more faith, more knowledge, and more strength to help her as best I could. I contacted every resource I could find to help her and help me be strong enough to help her. I asked all my friends and contacts to help make her dreams and wishes come true. I loved her more than I ever thought was possible. I taught her everything I felt she needed to know to make a beautiful transition home to our Heavenly Father.

My daughter loved me more than anyone else in the world. She adored me. I am so grateful that there was no one she would rather be with her than me. This past summer when my other children were struggling with their grief, with our new family dynamics without Celeste, when they pushed me away or wouldn't talk, their rejection would send my mind into a whirlwind.

I would grieve for the one child who adored me and wanted to be with me more than anyone. Why did she have to go? I would want to be with her more than anything else in the world. It was at those times I could hear her beautiful voice whisper in my heart and soul, "Mummy, I love you!"

My children have passed through those rough grief stages now. My youngest hugs me randomly every day and I continue to smother him with love and cherish each embrace. My oldest talks with me now more than ever, not necessarily about her feelings about her sister yet but about everything else under the sun. She seems more grateful for our time together and hugs me to say thanks each time. My middle child—he used to be third out of four, although I still tell everyone I have four children, one just happens to be in Heaven—is not quite up to talking yet and pulls 14-year-old attitude. However, he makes it quite known when we watch TV that he has reserved that space next to "Mother" as he maturely calls me now. It feels good to know he still needs and wants his Mummy too!

These are all new normals after three years of each day finding a new normal. That is what your life will be about, too. Finding normalcy in the craziness of this terrible disease.

It may seem impossible some days, but it's not. It's so important to find hope in every circumstance, no matter what happens.

Thank you for allowing us to share our journey and story of friendship and inspiration, of struggles and miracles, of joy and sadness, of love and loss, with you. Celeste is with me every day, and in her honor, we share *Two Mothers, One Prayer*.

Lorna Byrne in her book *A Message of Hope from the Angels* states:

> Hope makes the impossible possible. Strength is contagious and courage is doing what we never thought we could do, doing it despite the fear, despite the dread, despite the pain and heartache. Hope can be given to others. It gives us strength and courage and then hope grows.

May you find hope, strength, and courage. Please, reach out, connect, reflect, express, and love, no matter where your road leads you.

RECOMMENDED RESOURCES

Laura's Reading List

Aspire by Kevin Hall
A Message of Hope from the Angels by Lorna Byrne
Angels in my Hair by Lorna Byrne
Anticancer by David Servan-Schreiber
Daring Greatly by Brené Brown
Dreamhealer: A True Story of Miracle Healing by Adam McLeod
Dreamhealer 2: A Guide to Healing and Self-Empowerment by
    Adam McLeod
Getting well Again by Dr. Carl Simonton MD, Stephanie
    Matthews-Simonton, and James Creighton
The Anatomy of Hope by Dr. Gerome Groupman
The Biology of Belief by Bruce H. Lipton
The Gifts of Imperfection by Brené Brown
The Greatest Salesman in the World by Og Mandino
The Healing Codes by Dr. Alex Loyd and Dr. Ben Johnson
The Power of Intention by Wayne Dyer
The Spontaneous Healing of Belief by Gregg Braden
Today I Begin a New Life by Dave Blanchard
*Zero Limits: The Secret Hawaiian System for Wealth, Health, Peace
    and More* by Joe Vitale and Dr. Ihaleakala Hew Len

Laura's Emotional Toolbox

Emotional Freedom Technique (EFT)
    www.eftuniverse.com
Eye Movement Desensitization and Reprocessing (EMDR)
    www.emdr.com
Sedona Method
    www.sedona.com
The Emotion Code
    www.drbradleynelson.com
The Healing Code
    www.thehealingcodes.com
Therapeutic Touch (TT)
    www.therapeutic-touch.org

OUR GRATITUDE LIST!

We are so very grateful for so many wonderful people who have helped us over the last three years. Finishing the book would not have been possible without Kristen Eckstein, the ultimate book coach, and our fabulous editor Kelly Epperson. We are grateful to the wonderful team at the Enlightened Bestseller Mastermind Experience: Marci Schimoff, Geoff Affleck, Chris Attwood, and Janet Bray Attwood. We are grateful to all the wonderful people— doctors, nurses, social workers, authors, and fellow parents—who provided endorsements for the book. We are especially grateful to Kevin Hall for writing the foreword. Thank you!

We would like to publicly thank the special contributors to our Indiegogo Crowdsourcing campaign: Phil Cicio, Lina and Turner Larabie, Mechelle Scheuermann, Sabrina Martinez, Janet and Graham Schurman, Geoff Affleck, Ellen Rogin, Pleasantview Funeral Home & Cemetery, Helen Mattingly, Gaby Abdelgadir, Bryan L'Ecuyer, JoAnne Lane, Peter and Penny Johnson, Michael Ong, Kevin Bolibruck, Brian and Rita Duplessis.

Individually we would like to thank:

Laurie

I would like to thank my sisters—Aunt Cookie/Christie and Aunt D/Donna—for always being my rock and for allowing their children to home school with Hayley so she would not feel alone. Annika Sorenstam for being Hayley's celebrity friend to keep her spirits up. Megan for keeping Taylor and Matthew fed while we were in the hospital. Cynthia for coordinating meal lists during our hospital stay. Our families for their unending love and support. Dr. Minturn, Dr. Phillips, Dr. Hill-Kayser, and Dr. Goli for their compassion and individualized treatment plan to heal our Hayley.

G-Mal and G-Lynne for their support and kindness to Hayley and our whole family when we really needed it. Dee for her yummy brownies and treats and for being Hayley's adult friend and golf buddy who truly understands and listens.

Laura

My extraordinary business coach Lisa Peck who has held me together for the last three years. I don't know how I could have done it without all your support and guidance. My other lifeline was Vivian Cannataro, who was available at a moment's notice to help me get through the darkest hours. And Barbara Horne put me back together when it was all said and done. I had such wonderful spiritual leaders: Bishop Denis Tisi, Bishop Charles Baxter, Bishop Jeff Glanfield, President David Homer and his counselor Jeff Roy. My dear friend and native healer Karen McNaughton. Sick Kids Chaplain Ani J (Ani Jamyang Donma) and the wonderful team of Therapeutic Touch practitioners—Sally-Ann Kerman, Maureen Smith, Clare Stark, Christina, Sally, Heather, and Darka Neill—who came to the hospital week after week. I am so grateful for all the friends and family who supported us while Celeste was in hospital. Morticia and Chris for providing Matt and Grayson a place to stay multiple times. Lissa Joy for coming to the hospital and doing my laundry! Rachel for bringing bread and peanut butter and jam so I could make Celeste's favourite sandwiches. Dan for making the best chocolate cupcakes and coming at moment's notice to bring me yummy food when I couldn't get away. Tim and Mary for opening their home to me and letting me use their kitchen to make chicken couscous for Celeste. Leslie and Ruth for letting me crash for the night when I first arrived in Toronto. Doug for being there and taking me out for lunch. The missionaries who gave blessings and visited Celeste. All our wonderful nurses, and especially Linh, who made beautiful pictures of Winnie the Pooh for Celeste. Dr. Bartels, Dr. Doyle, Dr. Drake, Dr. Fischer, and Dr. Cairney. Debbie Berlin-Romalis for being so supportive and understanding. The incredible staff of Ronald McDonald House in Toronto. Greg Sentence for coming all the way to Toronto to visit and support Celeste. Lorie Gannon for sending me Zero Limits at the perfect time. Jack Canfield, Hale Dwoskin, Carol Look, Bob Proctor, Adam McLeod, Crystal Starr, and Kara at Nick Vujicic's office for all the support, advice, referrals and prayers. President Thomas S. Monson for meeting with Celeste and praying for her daily. Stuart McLean and Louise Curtiss at CBC, Andrina Turenne and Alexa Dirks from Chic Gamine and the staff at the AMC Theatre for all the wonderful gifts. Dale and Andrea at OWN Life Story Project for the wonderful interview and sending Celeste a copy. Natasha and David, Steph and Neil, JoAnne, and Melissa for watching Grayson at a moment's notice. Mark Boyd for covering for Matt at work. Hannah for taking care of our hamster. Lina, Sharon, and Claudia for painting Celeste's room. Trish for snow blowing our walk and driveway almost all winter. Terry and Mark for being our on-call paramedics. Lisa for finding us a wheelchair last minute and Lisa's neighbour who lent it to us for as long as we needed it. Kirsten for bringing makeup for the Celeste and Hayley and me. Alex Sears (Photos by Alex) and Ed Limon (PGP Studios) for photographing and filming the soup party. Tracey Cerisano, the Hamilton Stake Young Women, Welland Ward Young Women, and London Second Ward Young Women for all their support of Celeste. Julie for planning the Celestabration. All the students and staff of Saunders Secondary School and Tie Day. All the support from the Welland Relief Society and London Second Ward Relief Society for sending meals nightly for six weeks. Judy for opening her home to Matt, Grayson, and me for five weeks. Rick for bringing Celeste's dress from Toronto so she could see it. Fiz for writing such a beautiful song for Celeste. Marie, Marcus, Kelly, Joanna, Julia, Erika, Michele, Rita Carrey, and the staff of the BBC and the thousands of people who bombarded Hollywood with requests for Celeste. Lastly, the biggest thank you to David Tenant, Robin Williams, Jim Carrey, Celine Dion, Anne Hathaway, Karen Gillian, and Matt Smith for taking time out of your busy schedules to befriend Celeste in her last days. It meant so much to her and us. Thank you!

ABOUT THE AUTHORS

Laura Lane has worked with, trained with, and learned from the world's leaders in personal growth and development: Jack Canfield, Bob Proctor, Chris and Janet Attwood, Marci Schimoff, Steve Siebold, Stephen Covey, Kevin Hall, Ty Bennett, Dave Blanchard, and Wayne Dyer. She has been certified and trained as a LifeSuccess Consultant to teach and coach Bob Proctor's personal growth and development programs. She has also trained and certified as a Passion Test Facilitator to guide individuals and groups through the Passion Test Process developed by Chris and Janet Attwood. Laura is a published children's book author, poet, artist, speaker, coach, and gallery owner. She is the mother of four children: Desiree, Celeste, Connlan, and Grayson. Laura and her husband, Matt, currently reside in the Niagara Region of Ontario, Canada. Visit her website www.lauralane.ca to learn more about her various programs, current artistic and writing projects, and speaking engagements.

———————

Laurie Nersten is the mother of three wonderful teenaged children: Hayley, Matthew, and Taylor. As a family they love going to the beach and spending time with extended family. Laurie enjoys volunteering at Calvary Bible Church, assisting with the youth.

Laurie trained and worked in the information field but has dedicated the last four years to caring for Hayley and homeschooling between appointments and different treatment plans. Her strong Christian faith has helped her to keep focused on all of God's promises and remain positive. Laurie looks forward to the day she and her husband, Anthony, can spend quiet days by the lake. They currently reside in Hunterdon County, New Jersey.

CPSIA information can be obtained at www.ICGtesting.com
Printed in the USA
LVOW01s0457210415

435373LV00013B/122/P